Fusion Fitness

"Chan Ling offers a comprehensive guide to understanding how the body works, the effects of training and nutrition, plus analysis of such trendy topics as core stability. With clear diagrams and photos, this a very user-friendly manual for anyone looking to get the best from their work-outs."

— **Andrew Shields,** *Time Out London*

"The book incorporates the author's knowledge and understanding of Eastern teachings and combines them with fitness and health techniques of the West, creating a new fitness routine for modern day living; a fusion of ideas and disciplines. This is a book for people serious about health and fitness."

— **Hannah Green,** *Limited Edition*

"This book is ideal for those people who are looking to embark on a safe and holistic exercise programme while being able to understand underlying theory behind it. Fusion Fitness is a good read for people wanting to start an exercise regime from home, and especially for the over 50's, as the book has dedicated chapters to this age group."

— **Kerryn Samprey,** *Personal Trainer*

"*Fusion Fitness* demonstrates that both Eastern and Western approaches aim to achieve similar goals: coordination, core stability, flexibility, muscle strength, awareness of mind and body, and internal energy balance. This book combines theory and practice, explaining how exercises should be performed and why they are effective."

— *Health & Fitness Matters,* Harpers Fitness

To my mother, with love.

Ordering

Trade bookstores in the U.S. and Canada please contact:

Publishers Group West
1700 Fourth Street, Berkeley CA 94710
Phone: (800) 788-3123   Fax: (510) 528-3444

Hunter House books are available at bulk discounts for textbook course adoptions; to qualifying community, health-care, and government organizations; and for special promotions and fund-raising. For details please contact:

Special Sales Department
Hunter House Inc., PO Box 2914, Alameda CA 94501-0914
Phone: (510) 865-5282   Fax: (510) 865-4295
E-mail: sales@hunterhouse.com

Individuals can order our books from most bookstores, by calling
(800) 266-5592, or from our website at **www.hunterhouse.com**

Project Credits

Cover Design: Peri Poloni, Knockout Books
Book Production: Jil Weil / Hunter House
Copy Editor: Kelley Blewster
Proofreader: John David Marion
Indexer: Nancy D. Peterson
Acquisitions Editor: Jeanne Brondino
Editor: Alexandra Mummery
Publicity Coordinator: Earlita K. Chenault
Sales & Marketing Coordinator: Jo Anne Retzlaff
Customer Service Manager: Christina Sverdrup
Order Fulfillment: Lakdhon Lama
Administrator: Theresa Nelson
Computer Support: Peter Eichelberger
Publisher: Kiran S. Rana

Fusion Fitness

Combining the Best from East and West

Chan Ling Yap, Ph.D.

Foreword by STEPHANIE COOK

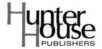

Hunter House
PUBLISHERS

First published in 2002 by A & C Black Publishers Ltd 37 Soho Square, London W1D 3QZ;
www.acblack.com

Hunter House Inc., Publishers
PO Box 2914
Alameda CA 94501-0914

Library of Congress Cataloging-in-Publication Data

Yap, Chan Ling, Ph.D.
Fusion fitness : combining the best from East and West / Chan Ling Yap ; foreword by Stephanie Cook.— 1st ed.
p. cm.
Originally published: London : A & C Black, 2002.
Includes bibliographical references and index.
ISBN 0-89793-378-8 (pbk.) — ISBN 0-89793-379-6 (cloth)
1. Exercise. 2. Nutrition. I. Title.
GV481 .Y36 2002
613.7′1—dc21   2002011971

Photo Credits

Photographs: Grant Pritchard
Medical illustrations: Peter Gardiner
Exercise drawings: Jean Ashley
Photo of t'ai chi session: Jimmy C. K. Lee
Photo of Fusion Fitness class: Tony Loftas
Models: Chan Ling Yap, Charlotte Steptoe, Christine Oliver, and Lee Webb

Manufactured in Canada by Transcontinental Printing

9 8 7 6 5 4 3 2 1   First Edition   03 04 05 06 07

Contents

List of Illustrations viii
    Tables and Sidebars . . . . *viii*
    Figures and Photos . . . . *ix*

Foreword xii

Preface xiv

Acknowledgments xvii

About the Author xvii

1   **Exercise, Past and Present** 1

2   **Getting Started: Fitness and Its Benefits for You** 5
    A Balanced Fitness Program 6
    Fitness Assessment and Testing 11
    Ready, Set, Go! 15

3   **Understanding Your Body and Its
Responses to Exercise** 17
    The Skeleton 17
    The Muscles 23
    The Respiratory System 37
    Energy and Energy Systems 40

4   **Setting Sensible Targets for Exercise** 46
    Body Shape or Somatotype 47
    Keeping the Body Ticking 49
    Food and Diet 51
    Spot Reduction of Fat 54
    Getting Older 55
    Gender Differences 56

5   **Fusion Fitness: The Broad Approach to Exercise** 58
    Holistic Regimes 60
    *Finding the Best Combination: The Art and Science
    of "Fusion" Exercise* 68

Contents

6 The Warm-Up: Getting Ready to Exercise **70**
What Is a Warm-Up? 70
The Benefits of a Warm-Up 74

7 Aerobic Training: Staying on the Curve **75**
Programming Effective Training: The Aerobic Curve 76
Different Kinds of Aerobic Training 78
Avoiding Overtraining 84

8 Body Conditioning: Training for Strength and Endurance . **85**
Basic Principles of Muscle Contraction 86
Training Using Body Resistance: The Fusion Recipe 90

9 Fusion Exercises: Putting Theory into Practice **99**
Lower Torso and Legs 102
Upper Torso and Arms 132

10 Training for Flexibility: Eliminating Stress and Strain **141**
The Benefits of Stretching 142
Types of Stretching 143
Training Exercises for Flexibility 147
The Torso 148
The Arms 154
The Buttocks and Legs 154
The Thigh, Shin, and Calf Muscles 157
Progression in Training 160
Relaxation 163

11 Sports and Exercise Injuries and Training to Avoid Them . **165**
Common Sports Injuries 165
Safe Training 168
Treatment for Sports Injuries 173

12 Nutrition: The Other Side of the Fitness Equation **174**
Balancing Food Requirements 175
Present Dietary Patterns 186
Dietary Intake for Sports 188
Minerals 193
Vitamins 198
Water 204
Alcohol 205

13 Exercise and Eating for People over 50 . . . . **207**
  Aerobics: Keep On Moving! 208
  Strength, Endurance, and Stretching 209
  Nutrition for Changing Needs 222

Appendix 1: Calculating Basal Metabolic Rate (BMR) **227**

Appendix 2: Calories and Joules: An Explanation **229**

Appendix 3: Training Programs **230**
  Program 1 (1 hour) 230
  Program 2 (1 hour) 232
  Program 3 (1 hour) 234
  Program 4 (1 hour) 237
  Program 5 (20 minutes) 239

Notes **242**

Bibliography **243**

Additional Resources: Selected Useful Websites **245**

Index **246**

List of Illustrations

Tables and Sidebars

Chapter 1
Women in the Olympic Games 3

Chapter 2
Perceived Rates of Exertion 9
Sample Screening Questionnaire 10
Determining Your Body Mass Index
    (BMI) 12
World Health Organization's Classifica-
    tion of Blood Pressure 14

Chapter 3
The Spinal Column 19
The Skeletal Muscles of the Body 27
The Heart and Circulatory System 36
The Cardiac Cycle and Hypertension . . . 38
A Comparison of Energy Systems 44

Chapter 4
Caloric Content of Selected Foods and
    Duration of Activities Required for
    their Utilization 52
Average Energy Expended in Everyday
    Activities and Selected Sports 53
Average BMR, RDA in the U.S., and
    EAR of Energy in the U.K., by
    Gender/Age 54

Chapter 7
Effective Personal-training Zones 77

Chapter 8
Selected Major Opposing-muscle
    Groups 89
How Does Fusion Fitness Differ from
    Pilates? 97

Chapter 11
Selected Major Sports and Exercise
    Injuries 169

Chapter 12
What Counts as One Serving? 176
Foods Rich in Carbohydrates 177
Foods and Their Cholesterol
    Content 180
Foods that Lower Blood
    Cholesterol 180
Blood Cholesterol Levels and Their
    Associated Risk Factors 180
Improving Protein Intake from Animal
    and Plant Sources 185
Total Daily Energy Intakes Required
    for Intensive Training in a Number
    of Different Competitive Sports 189
Glycemic Index for Selected Foods . . . 190
Carbohydrate Intake During Training
    for Competition 190
Recommended Daily Intake of Macro-
    minerals and Microminerals 192
Recommended Daily Intake of
    Vitamins 202

Chapter13
Some Beneficial Foods for Seniors 225

Figures and Photos

Chapter 2

Box Push-ups 6
Full-floor Push-ups 6
Training with Weights 6
Step Test 15
Sit-and-Reach Test 16
Hamstring Test 16
Shoulder Test 16
Quadriceps Test 16

Chapter 3

The Body's Framework 18
The Spinal Column 19
Main Types of Joints 22
The Structure of the Ball-and-Socket
    Joint in the Hip 23
The Principal Skeletal Muscles of
    the Body 24
Biceps and Triceps: Extension and
    Flexion of Muscles and How They
    Work in Support of Each Other 26
The Bundles of Muscle Fibers that
    Make Up the Striated or Skeletal
    Muscles 31
Actin and Myosin: How Muscles
    Work 32
Motor Nervous System 33
The Heart and Circulatory System 36
How We Breathe 39
The Energy Cycle 42

Chapter 4

The Three Basic Body Shapes 48

Chapter 5

Shoulder Stand 61
Headstand 61
The Plow Pose 61
Back Arch Pose 61
The Peacock Pose 63
The Dog Pose 63
Open-air Participation in T'ai Chi 65

Chapter 6

Mobilizing the Hips, Trunk, and
    Shoulders 71
Mobilizing the Ankle, Knee, and Hips . . 71
Stretching the Calf Muscles 72
Stretching the Adductor Muscles in
    the Inner Thigh and Hamstring 72
Stretching the Deltoid and the
    Triceps 73
Stretching the Quadriceps 73

Chapter 7

Aerobic Training Curves 77
Low-impact and Low-intensity
    Movements 80
The Grapevine 81
Side Lunge, Knee Lifts, and
    Heel Digs 81
High-impact Movements 82
Aerobic Circuit Training with Step
    and Nonstep Stations 83

Chapter 8

Types of Muscle Contractions 87
Muscle Contractions in Sit-ups 88

List of Illustrations

The Iliopsoas: Stabilizing the Hips
and Lower Back 93
The Transversospinalis-Multifidus 93
Neutral Body Alignment 96
Stabilizing the Core 96
The Evolution of Fusion Fitness 98

Chapter 9

The Structure of the Abdominal
Muscles 102
The Conventional Body Crunch 103
Transverse Abdominal Squeeze 105
Reverse Abdominal Squeeze 107
Reverse Abdominal Squeeze,
Legs Straight 108
Moon Walk I 109
Moon Walk II 109
Side Reaches 110
Shoulder to Knee 111
"Z" Position 112
Erector Spinae: The Principal Back
Muscle 113
Back Extension 114
The Principal Muscles in the Buttocks
and Upper Thigh 115
Back Leg Lift 116
Side Leg Lift 117
Straight-back Leg Extension 118
Right-angle Lift 119
Acute Angle Moving in 120
Modified Buttock Lift 121
Inner Thigh Muscles: Adductors 122
Inner Thigh Seesaw: Toning the
Inner Thigh 123
The Upper Thigh Muscles:
Quadriceps 124
Conventional Squats 125
Ski Squats 125
Travel Squats 125

Pedal and Stride 126
The Barre 128
The Hamstring: The Muscles at the
Back of the Thigh 129
Leg Curl 130
The Calf and Shin Muscles 131
Heel Raises and Heel Digs 131
The Chest Muscles: Pectoralis Major
and Minor 132
Push-ups 132
The Chest Press 134
The Muscles Between the Shoulder
Blades: Trapezius and Rhomboids . . 135
The Latissimus Dorsi: Muscles Stretching
from Spine to Upper Arm 135
The Three Principal Muscles in the Arm:
Deltoid, Biceps, Triceps 136
Upright Row for the Deltoid, Biceps Curl,
and Triceps Extension 137
Triceps Extension on the Floor 138
Back Arm Lifts 139
Scissoring the Arms 140

Chapter 10

An Imbalance in Muscle Strength
and Flexibility 142
A Shortened Iliotibial Band 143
Ballistic Stretch: Inner Thigh
(Adductors) 144
Static Stretching for the Hamstring . . . 145
Active Stretching for the Hamstring . . . 145
Stretching the Hamstring with Help . . . 146
Feline Stretch 148
Prayer Position 149
Half Serpent 149
Full Serpent 150
Full Cobra 151
The Yawn 151
"Z" Stretch 152

The Roll-Back *153*
The Roll-Forward *153*
Forearm Twist *154*
Buttocks Stretch *155*
Hold the Horns *155*
Groin Stretch *156*
Wide-angle Stretch *157*
Thigh and Shin-muscle Stretch *158*
Forward-bend Stretch *158*
Full Wide-angle Stretch *160*
Stretching in Flight *161*
Full Flight *162*

Chapter 11
Injuries to the Foot Tendons *167*
Injuries to the Knee Ligament *168*
Extreme Knee Flexion *172*
Deep Knee Squat *172*
Poorly Executed "V" Sit-up and
    Full-length Push-up *173*

Chapter 12
Food Guide Pyramid *175*
Pathways of High- and Low-density
    Lipoproteins in the Body *183*

Chapter 13
Scaling the Wall *211*
Wall Walk *212*
Feline Stretch *214*
Standing Feline Stretch *215*
Squats with Support *216*
Thigh Stretch with Support *217*
Back Leg Lift *218*
Leg Curls *219*
Side Leg Lift *219*
Calf Stretch Using Wall *221*
Hamstring Stretch Using Wall *221*
A 50+ Exercise Class in Action *223*

Foreword

Sports and exercise are an integral part of many people's lives. More women than ever before are benefiting from exercise, not just in fitness regimes but in competitive sports as well. For example, the Sydney Olympics in 2000 marked the first time that women had the chance to compete in modern pentathlon, even though the event was introduced into the Olympic Games in 1912 by the founder of the modern Olympic movement, Baron Pierre de Coubertin. In winning an Olympic gold medal I reached a pinnacle that few people ever achieve, but you do not have to compete at an Olympic Games to appreciate many of the benefits that exercise can bring to your life. *Fusion Fitness* is designed to improve the health and fitness of both men and women, encouraging them to play a more active role in improving their health and lifestyles and in increasing their understanding of important issues.

The very nature of modern pentathlon, with its five diverse disciplines of shooting, fencing, swimming, show jumping, and running, embodies the idea of the fusion of different sports and the necessity of a balanced approach. Through training for all these events I have come to learn the benefits of cross training. In a similar way, this book integrates the best from a wide range of exercise and fitness techniques, with input from different cultures around the world.

I have always led a very active life and am thankful for the good health and fitness that I enjoy. I have been very fortunate in having had the opportunity to participate in a range of different sports from a young age, and I have competed internationally at both cross-country running and modern pentathlon. At school I was no remarkable athlete, but I enjoyed a variety of sports from hockey to tennis to track and field. It was not until I was studying medicine at Cambridge University that I took sports in any way seriously, when I was selected to row for the university women's lightweight crew.

Through my medical studies I became particularly interested in the ways the human body adapts to exercise and in the importance of having a sound scientific basis—along with a careful nutritional plan—behind any training regime. The explanations of exercise and fitness contained in *Fusion Fitness* are based firmly in modern medical and scientific knowledge. The reader is able to understand the derivation of certain exercises, thereby encouraging the accurate accomplishment of them and helping to prevent injury.

My life has been enriched in many different ways by sports and exercise and the consequences of being fit and healthy. From a very early age, exercise provides a fun way for children to develop social skills and learn the importance of teamwork. This social element continues into adulthood, with many a lifelong friendship being built through shared experiences, whether through competitive sports, attending exercise classes, or recreational jogging. Exercise is a vital means of improving your health and well-being and also serves to improve confidence levels through looking good and feeling good about yourself. It also provides a great way to reduce stress levels, and the fitter you are, the more energy you have for other activities, as well. If you integrate some form of exercise into your daily routine, the positive effects will extend into all areas of your life.

Fusion Fitness goes a step beyond many other books in the field by addressing the needs of both fitness instructors and students, as well as appealing to a wider general audience. The author is established as a specialist in the field of health and fitness, and this book reflects the wealth of experience she has to offer. It provides a reliable source of information that is clearly presented, easy to understand, and yet technically accurate. This book constitutes a major contribution towards the body of literature on health and fitness and fills a vital gap in the market.

— Stephanie Cook, MBE, BM, BCh (Oxon), MA (Cantab)
Modern Pentathlon Olympic Gold Medallist, Sydney 2000
Modern Pentathlon European and World Champion 2001

Preface

To have good health and to be fit is a blessing. A blessing, however, is not necessarily a right. Knowledge about how the human body works, a balanced diet, and regular exercise are vital to fitness and health.

When I first took up exercise, I went into it unquestioningly. I did what I was instructed to do because I was told that it would be good for me. There was little explanation offered as to why. I might be told, "This is to improve the shape of your legs." But I wanted to know why, in what way, and how! Later, as the number of available exercise regimes multiplied and different methods of improving body shape and fitness grew, so did the confusion of ideas and methods, each one claiming to be better than the others, and, even worse, claiming that the others were wrong.

My first exposure to the science of exercise came when I enrolled for a fitness instructor's course on exercising to music. I learned a lot, but my need to know more and my efforts to acquire knowledge beyond that needed to pass exams were frequently frustrated by the lack of information that was available. I am convinced that people have a right to know more about their body, how it works, and why they should exercise in a particular way. This, I believe, places considerable responsibility on instructors who, like other health and sports professionals, should have a wider and deeper understanding of the body than many often do. With improved technology in all aspects of our life, and with a more educated general public, surely there should also be improved knowledge of the body. We should be aware of how and why we are asked to exercise or move in a certain way, and of what fitness and nutrition can do for us.

In the field of competitive sports, much headway has been made. In the widely available books on running, for example, the training regimes offered are well grounded in science. I was impressed with the book *Keep On Running*, by Eric Newsholme, Tony Leech, and Glenda Duester.[1] It addresses the science of training and performance and explains the whys and wherefores of training methods. Most serious runners I have met know about muscles and the rationale and science behind their training regimes. That same knowledge is less common when I speak to people attending fitness and exercise classes. Most attendees place great reliance on the instructor's knowledge, and seem to unquestioningly accept what is taught. This may be because such classes are not competitive; the lack of a focus on winning results in a relaxed attitude about what participants are told to do. Nonetheless, the exercises that people perform in classes have an important impact on their health.

The implicit trust placed in fitness instructors and personal trainers must be backed up by the knowledge that what is being practiced is sound. I also believe that the boundaries of rigid disciplines—boundaries that are determined as much in the interests of commercialism as for the good of participants—can and should be crossed. While most disciplines have something to offer, not everything offered is either safe or beneficial. Integration of the most successful elements from the various disciplines is, I believe, the best way forward.

Fusion Fitness: Combining the Best from East and West aims to accomplish this goal. It is written for educators, fitness instructors, students in sports, and a general audience interested in exercise and how to stay fit. It contains information about exercise and nutrition, the body, and how it works. It takes the reader stage by stage through all the elements of fitness, from discussing the importance of cardiovascular conditioning, muscle strength, tone, and body shape, to looking at endurance and energy levels, flexibility, acquisition of motor skills, and avoiding injury. It offers an overview of human anatomy and physiology, especially as they relate to exercise and activity. It helps the reader adopt realistic goals for a fitness program. It examines several different exercise regimes popular today—from the ancient, such as yoga, to the modern, such as the Alexander Technique and Pilates—and explains the theory and practice behind combining the best of these into a system I call "fusion" exercise.

The book's central chapters are devoted to in-depth descriptions and illustrations of many warm-up, strength-building, and stretching techniques, organized to focus in turn on each muscle group. Many of the exercises are original and devised especially for this volume. Exercise and anatomy are not treated as separate fields of knowledge; for each set of exercises the relevant muscles and bones are identified and their functions explained, as are the reasons for adopting the recommended body alignments. By showing anatomically what can and cannot be achieved, I dispel many myths of the "miracles" attached to exercise. I have also included a detailed chapter on nutrition, and a special chapter for people over age 50.

Fusion Fitness is based on over twenty years' experience as a participant and, in more recent years, as an instructor in a wide variety of health and fitness classes. I have brought together my knowledge of a wide range of disciplines, choosing only the best and the safest elements from them to produce a "fusion exercise regime" for health and fitness. There is still further to go and there are improvements to be made, but the future of fusion fitness looks promising. I hope this book will be a positive step towards encouraging the practice of informed and holistic exercise.

Acknowledgments

I would like to thank my husband, Tony Loftas, for the encouragement, support, and help he has given me in writing the book. His background as a science writer and editor made his comments invaluable. Thanks go also to my children, Hsu Min and Lee, for their understanding and support. Lee deserves a special mention for his patience in teaching me the software that I used for the initial drawing of the diagrams and figures. I would also like to thank my students for their interest and encouragement. My thanks go to Charlotte Steptoe, Christine Oliver, and Lee Webb for helping in the demonstration of the exercises. I would also like to thank Stephanie Cook for taking the word of my daughter, a fellow runner, that this was a serious book and agreeing to read the manuscript and write the foreword. Finally, I would like to thank the staff of Hunter House, especially Alex Mummery and Kelley Blewster, for their discerning editing and production of the book.

About the Author

Chan Ling Yap, after obtaining a Ph.D. in the United Kingdom in 1973, returned to the University of Malaya to teach. In 1978 she joined the Food and Agriculture Organization of the United Nations in Rome, where she remained for 19 years. While in Rome, she explored a range of fitness regimes. The international nature of her work brought her into contact with fitness disciplines from many parts of the world and their underlying philosophies and ideas. As a person of Chinese extraction, she also has knowledge of Eastern practices; her mother was guided for many years by a master of Chinese martial arts. Following the family's return to the United Kingdom in 1997, she combined her knowledge of Eastern teachings and Western sports science to develop a new regime, Fusion Fitness.

Important Note

The material in this book is intended to provide a review of information regarding exercise and fitness. Every effort has been made to provide accurate and dependable information, and the contents of this book have been compiled through professional research and in consultation with medical professionals. However, always consult with a doctor or physical-therapy practitioner before undertaking a new exercise regimen or doing any of the exercises or following any of the suggestions contained in this book.

The author, publisher, and editors, and the professionals quoted in the book cannot be held responsible for any error, omission, or dated material in the book. The author and publisher are not liable for any damage or injury or other adverse outcome of applying the information in this book in an exercise program carried out independently or under the care of a licensed trainer or practitioner. If you have questions concerning the application of the information described in this book, consult a qualified and trained professional.

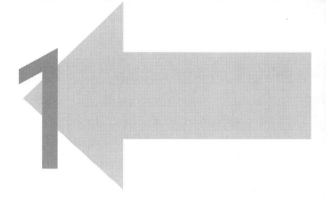

Exercise, Past and Present

Individuals have long used exercise to improve health and maintain physical fitness. The practice of yoga, which combines physical and mental disciplines to still the mind and body, dates back to prehistoric India. Records of ancient Chinese civilizations abound with examples of martial-art forms for improving mental discipline and physical prowess. In the martial arts, as in yoga, physical discipline is enmeshed with meditation and breath control. In Greek and Roman civilizations, pride of place was given to excellence in a wide range of sports. In ancient Greece, home of the Olympic Games, fitness and beauty of the human form were revered, and a regime of strict physical discipline was entrenched in the social structure of free-born Greeks, particularly the ruling class.

In the past, athletic activities fell almost entirely within the domain of men. It was generally men who hunted or fought on behalf of the family or state. Consequently, they were the ones most concerned with honing the necessary skills. Even in the disciplines that involved meditation and prayer, men were the main participants. The original sites of many martial-art forms in China were the monasteries. In ancient India, gurus in yoga practices were predominantly men.

Historically, women's role in the home and in the wider society did not encourage the pursuit of, or reverence for, physical activity per se. A few examples exist of lady ninjas in the period of the shoguns' rule in Japan; in Britain, Queen Boadicea is seen as the prototypical female warrior; and in ancient China there are stories of female acrobats with martial skills. Such women are exceptions to the rule. The higher up in the social structure, the greater was the propensity to regard women as adornments. Jewelry, dress, and makeup, rather than athletic skills, played a central role in beauty; the acquisition of the genteel arts of music, painting, and embroidery were seen as all important for the well-bred woman. This demarcation between men and women resulted in a concept of beauty wherein muscles and a toned body were admired in men but not in women. The "ideal" female form was rounder and softer.

This long-held perception of beauty still lingers today in some societies and cultures, but on the whole the twentieth century has witnessed a profound change in what represents feminine beauty. Industrial development and the inclusion of women in the workforce, together with emancipation, have been the engines of this change. Work outside the home provided women with income. What they should and could do—and how they looked and dressed—altered as they adapted to a new way of life determined increasingly by themselves. Medical advances, including control over fertility, and improved lay knowledge of what constitutes good health have provided additional stimulus to the evolution of a new definition of beauty. Out went the idea that physical helplessness meant femininity. Leanness is preferred to rotundity as people realize the adverse impact on health of being overweight. Even in the case of makeup, radical changes have taken place, with more emphasis on effects that reflect health.

Today, globalization has blurred the definition of what constitutes beauty. Beauty is increasingly equated with good health and fitness. Now all men and women can be beautiful: To feel beautiful is to be so. Feeling beautiful comes from within and touches upon everything a person does. It is the ability to exert control over the body, to move well and painlessly, to perform daily tasks efficiently and effectively. In brief, it is to be fit.

Today, both men and women pursue and participate equally in athletic events. Nowhere is this seen more clearly than in the Olympics. When the Olympics were first celebrated in Greece in 776 B.C., women were not allowed to participate, either as competitors or as spectators. It was not until 1900, in Paris, that women first participated at the Olympics and then only in golf and lawn tennis. In 1908, in London, just 36 women took part out of a total of over 2,000 athletes. The first postwar Olympics, held in London in 1948, had 385 women competitors out of a total of 4,000 athletes. Twenty years later the number had risen to 800, just 12 percent of the competitors. By the 2000 Olympic Games, in Sydney, Australia, the number of women had risen to

3,906, 38 percent of the total number of competitors (see below). Equally significant are the many events now open to women, which include the modern pentathlon, weight lifting, hammer, pole vault, and water polo.

Unfortunately, the advances in sports science and training regimes do not appear to have influenced the general public to any great extent. While virtually everyone appears to agree on the importance of being fit, relatively few people exercise regularly or pursue physical activity of any sort. We have a strange paradox whereby, parallel to ever greater high-level athletic achievement, the population at large has probably never been so lacking in fitness.

The Allied Dunbar National Fitness Survey, published in the United Kingdom in 1992, indicated that one in six people led a sedentary life.[2] These people had not undertaken a physical activity continuously for more than 20 minutes in the previous four weeks. Slightly over 30 percent of men and two-thirds of women had difficulties walking up a gentle slope at a moderate pace of three miles per hour. This finding, in smaller proportions, extended even to individuals between 16 and 24 years of age. Perhaps even more alarming were the numbers, even among the relatively young, who had difficulties in performing ordinary activities such as getting up from a couch and walking up the stairs.

More recent findings of the increasing number of people who are obese and the number of young people abusing alcohol add little optimism for an improvement in the malaise that seems to have gripped the population at large. The American Heart

Women in the Olympic Games			
	Male competitors	Female competitors	Total
Atlanta 1996	7,061	3,683	10,744
Sydney 2000	6,416	3,906	10,321
Change in percent	−9	+6	−4
Individuals' medal tally (2000 Olympics):			
Gold	103	56	159
Silver	38	42	80
Bronze	21	21	42

The progress of women in the Olympic Games reflects a changing emphasis among women in favor of fitness and competitive sports.

Association reports that only 22 percent of American adults get enough exercise to achieve cardiovascular fitness. As many as 250,000 deaths per year in the United States—about 12 percent of total deaths—are attributed to a lack of regular physical activity.[3] For many, pursuit of the lean look means special diets and even starvation rather than sensible exercise. The results can be anorexia, bulimia, and vacillating weight losses and gains.

The contrast between the progress made in competitive sports and the fitness level of the general public results from a number of causes. Probably chief among them is a misconception of what exercise entails. Many think that exercise is a vigorous physical activity that has to be pursued separately and is therefore ruled out by work commitments, children, and economic as well as time constraints. This is certainly inaccurate. Exercise is simply any activity that involves the use of muscles and increases the metabolism of the body. It can be easily incorporated into daily life. Moreover, if exercise is pursued for health, moderation rather then vigor is often the answer: Brisk walks may be a better option than running or even jogging.

Exercise includes a wide range of activities; it is not synonymous with sports. However, both for fitness instructors seeking to give their best and for students of exercise wanting to benefit the most, a basic education about health and fitness is vital. Understanding the different forms of exercise and the different components of fitness is important in designing and selecting the exercise program best suited to you. Knowing what your exercise aims are and what different exercises can do is also important.

You need to know how your body works, what it needs, what fitness means, and how to achieve it. What are the benefits of the different fitness components and exercise regimes? What can be achieved and what cannot be changed? How do you systematically exercise your muscles? How can you tackle common "problem areas," such as a flabby stomach? In the search for solutions I have taken a "fusion" approach, selecting and combining the best from East and West, to provide a balanced exercise regime that meets the present-day needs for fitness and for release from the stress of modern life. Last but not least, I have restored the place of eating and enjoying a varied diet to where it belongs in the spectrum of fitness and health.

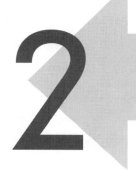

Getting Started: Fitness and Its Benefits for You

At its simplest, fitness means having the capacity to perform activities without exhaustion. This capacity, often taken for granted when young, is not easy to maintain throughout life. Fitness involves five elements:

- **strength** to provide the force needed for pushing, lifting, pulling, walking, running, and similar activities

- **endurance** to maintain effort long enough to finish a task and even go on to others

- **flexibility** to attain or maintain the full range of movements that the body should be able to do, such as twisting, bending, and reaching

- **motor skills** to enable the body to respond efficiently and effectively to external stimulus

- **circulatory (cardiovascular)** and **respiratory efficiency** to sustain these activities and for recovery after such efforts

A Balanced Fitness Program

A well-balanced program should include training components for the achievement of these five goals. If a particular fitness program does not cover all of them, it should be complemented with activities necessary to provide the balance.

To increase **strength** requires working with resistance, which can be provided using your own body or weights. In floor push-ups, for example, the resistance or weight is provided by the body. The level of resistance can be adjusted to meet personal needs and capacity. Push-ups from a kneeling position involve less resistance than if they are carried out with straight legs pivoting on the toes.

Strength development with body resistance (see illustrations): box push-ups (figure A) provide less body resistance than full-floor push-ups (figure B), in which the arm and chest muscles take on the full weight of the body. Strength development with weights (figure C): the heavier the weights, the greater the resistance.

Endurance is built up by increasing the number of repetitions and hence the duration of an activity.

Improving **flexibility** involves both stretching muscles and mobilizing the joints. When stretching the hamstring, for example, the knee joint is mobilized; stretching the inner thigh muscles mobilizes the hip joint.

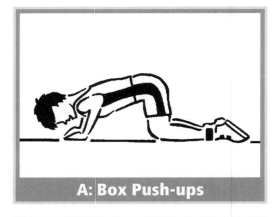

A: Box Push-ups

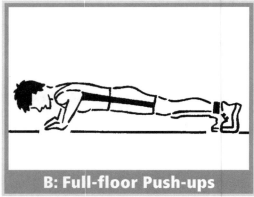

B: Full-floor Push-ups

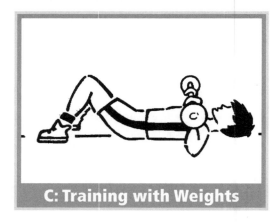

C: Training with Weights

Improvement in **motor skills** comes from practice. Generally, exercises performed in a class, such as aerobics, step, and line dancing, provide a good forum for their development because participants have to follow the instructor. Initially, the student's responses may be slow, but these should improve with experience because the body can be trained to move in a coordinated manner in response to signals received from the brain. Exercise trains the eye and the nervous network to be alert. The development of motor skills is often neglected, which is unfortunate since they decline with age. Motor skills can only be maintained if nerve cells receive repeated stimulation. Sports that encourage motor skill and reflex development include boxing, fencing, tennis, badminton, and karate or tae kwon do.

A structured **cardiovascular** workout is essential. Effected primarily through aerobic activities, it should aim to raise the heart rate gradually from its resting rate to one above normal. The heart is a muscular organ. Like any muscle it can be strengthened by being exercised and put to work. But herein lies the tricky part. How hard should it be made to work?

At rest, the pulse or heart rate of an average person measures around 60 to 70 beats per minute. Theoretically, the maximum heart rate that a normal healthy person could work toward is 220 minus his/her age. This is known as the *personal maximum heart rate*. In other words, if you are 40 years old, then your personal maximum

heart rate would be 180 beats per minute. However, if you have not done any sports before or have not exercised for some time—even if only because you were on a leisurely vacation for a couple of weeks—this number must be substantially moderated. In such a case, it would be advisable to work towards 60 percent of the personal maximum heart rate; for a 40-year-old, this means starting with a target heart rate of about 110 beats per minute. Over several weeks of regular training three to four times a week, this could be gradually raised to no more than 80 percent of the personal maximum heart rate, in this case, around 145 beats per minute (see the section on energy systems in Chapter 3).

A different method, called the Karvonen formula, is used in the United States to determine the target heart rate. In this formula, the resting heart rate is deducted from the personal maximum heart rate. This gives the reserve heart rate. Multiply this number by the intensity at which you wish to work, and add the result to the resting heart rate. Let's again use the example of a 40-year-old:

- Personal maximum heart rate:
  $220 - 40 = 180$

- Reserve heart rate (assuming a resting heart rate of 70): $180 - 70 = 110$

- Target heart rate if training at 60 percent intensity: $(110 \times 0.60) + 70 = 136$

- Target heart rate if training at 70 and 80 percent intensity: 147 and 158 respectively

To achieve the most effectiveness, the recommended aerobic training zone is normally 60 to 80 percent of the personal maximum heart rate. Working below 60 percent is of little use, and working above 80 percent causes fatigue to set in rapidly.

Very rarely, unless training for specific competitive sports, would anyone be encouraged to work towards their personal maximum heart rate. Instead, it is preferable, with increased fitness, to increase the duration of the workout within the same training zone. It is important to note that with increased fitness, the heartbeat is not raised as much by a given intensity of work. Thus, for the individual to reach the same training heart rate, he/she will have to intensify the workout. As a result, as fitness increases, maintaining training within 60 and 80 percent of the personal maximum heart rate automatically involves an increase in effort.

A good workout is always based on the principle of overload, that is, giving the body more work and exertion than it is accustomed to, in order to improve fitness. Thus, the greater the fitness the greater the load. Inevitably, there should be some feeling of increased exertion. How much, as illustrated above, can be indicated by taking one's pulse rate. This is easy enough when working on the treadmill or the bicycle, but can be difficult in a class situation. A general guideline in this instance is to work toward a comfortable level, where you are breathing hard without being breathless or giddy, and are able to continue the same level of effort. This is referred to as the *perceived exertion rate*, a scale developed by Gunner Borg (see table on page 9). The perceived exertion rate is a convenient measure for those on medication or with unusually high or low resting heart rates, where the pulse rate is a less reliable indicator of effort.

According to this scale, the rank 6–7, or "somewhat hard," is the minimum you should aim for in order to work aerobically. If perceived exertion is at 10–11, or "very hard," you should slow down. If at any point you feel that you have reached this stage, moderate your workout. Walk briskly instead of jogging, leave out any bouncy or high-impact moves, reduce the vigor of arm movements, but do not stop. An abrupt halt at the peak of the workout would lead to a

A note of caution: These levels of exertion are only guidelines. It is much more important that you feel comfortable, without any sense of giddiness, pain, or forced exertion. A great deal of sensible judgement is required. No one but the individual involved can fine-tune his/her own fitness program.

Perceived Rates of Exertion

Categories of exertion	Perceived exertion by rank
None	0
Extremely light	1
Quite light	2–3
Moderate	4–5
Somewhat hard	6–7
Hard	8–9
Very hard	10–11
Extremely hard	12
Maximum exertion	13

"pooling" of blood as the workout on the calf muscles stops. This reduces the return of blood to the heart, which in turn reduces the amount of blood that can be pumped to the rest of the body, and results in giddiness or even fainting.

In all workouts, whether in a class or on your own, even when jogging in the countryside, always start with a warm-up. This should consist of movements to mobilize the joints, ensuring that the synovial fluid that cushions them is warm and giving the lubrication necessary to ease their movements. A warm-up also gradually prepares the muscles, ligaments, and tendons for the increased exertion that is to follow. Then do a preparatory stretch. As the word suggests, this stretch prepares the body for bigger and possibly more vigorous movements in the main workout. These prepara-

tory stretches help reduce the incidence of sports injury, which can occur if the body is launched into vigorous activity without sufficient preparation.

On completion of the workout, again stretch all the muscles that have been involved, paying special attention to the hamstrings and the inner thigh muscles, holding them longer than in a preparatory stretch.

Muscles shorten with age, especially with sustained muscle contractions, as is inevitable in any workout and even in daily activities. Left unattended, shortened muscles—especially the hamstring and the back muscles—can give rise to poor posture and the bent frame commonly associated with aging. Stretching at the end of a workout also helps reduce muscle aches; it maintains the flexibility needed for ordinary day-to-day activities such as bending to tie shoelaces, soaping the back, reaching up, and twisting. The reduction in muscle tightness and the greater mobility of joints that accompany stretches contribute significantly to reducing accidents that cause injury and breakage of bones.

Finally, before embarking on any program of fitness, it is advisable to undergo a medical checkup and a fitness test. The major issues that should be addressed are listed in the screening questionnaire I use for my Fusion Fitness classes (sample on page 10). This kind of questionnaire is usually completed when joining a fitness club

Sample Screening Questionnaire

Name: _____ Age: _____ Female _____ Male _____

Address (Home): _____ Phone _____

Address (Office): _____ Phone _____

Person to be contacted in case of accident: _____

Phone (Home): _____ Phone (Office): _____

Please answer the following questions (check appropriate box or boxes)

1. If you already exercise regularly, please describe type and frequency of exercise.

   _____

	No	Yes/Unsure*
2. Have you ever had any injury, illness, or back or joint condition that may be aggravated by vigorous exercise?	____	____
3. Have you ever had: arthritis, asthma, diabetes, epilepsy, hernia, dizziness, gout, circulation problems, or an ulcer?	____	____
4. Has your mother, father, brother, or sister had any heart problem prior to age 60?	____	____
5. Have you ever had a heart condition, high blood pressure, rheumatic fever, stroke, high cholesterol, palpitations, murmurs, or chest pains?	____	____
6. Are you now or have you recently been pregnant? If yes, please state number of months into or since pregnancy: _____ months.	____	____
7. Are you taking any medicine prescribed by a medical practitioner?	____	____

*If you have answered any questions with yes/unsure, you should check with your doctor before starting any exercise program. **Please note:** You are responsible for your own health and safety. Should your health status change, please seek medical advice and inform me.

What benefits do you want from exercise? (Please check appropriate item(s).)

___ Weight management   ___ Improved cardiovascular fitness   ___ Social enjoyment

___ Improved muscle tone   ___ Improve or maintain overall fitness   ___ Good health

Others (please specify) _____

General advice on exercise

1. Do not eat for at least two hours before exercise.
2. Drink moderate quantities of water throughout the workout.
3. Wear appropriate footwear and clothing.
4. Work out at a sensible pace; to improve fitness, exercise at least three times per week.

I have completed the Fusion Fitness Screening Questionnaire and I understand the advice and accept the conditions detailed above.

Signed _____ Date _____

or center. The objective is to establish if there are any problems that might require referral to a medical service for clearance before starting an exercise program. If you have an instructor or trainer, keep him/her informed of any medical problems or injury, even after you have completed the questionnaire. It is important to discuss your needs and objectives with your instructor.

Fitness Assessment and Testing

Many fitness clubs ask new participants to undergo fitness testing. Fitness testing is simply a means to establish a baseline from which a person embarking on an exercise regime can work and progress. It also gauges health, already covered to some extent by the screening questionnaire, and fitness. In addition to establishing height, weight, body fat, resting pulse rate, and blood pressure, tests for strength, stamina/ endurance, and flexibility are also usually conducted. The tests conducted vary in complexity depending on the activity to be pursued. The following are some of the measures most commonly used to assess fitness.

Weight, Height, and Body Mass Index

The measurement of weight and height has traditionally been used to gauge whether a person deviates from the "ideal body weight" and whether weight loss or weight gain should be pursued. In the past, weight/height tables established by life-insurance companies were used to determine what was "normal." However, comparing an individual's weight and height to a life-insurance table was only broadly indicative of whether he or she was overweight. This is because the weight/height tables failed to reveal one's body composition, that is, his/her ratio of muscle to fat. Since muscle weighs more than fat, weighing more does not necessarily indicate excess weight. Furthermore, since the tables were computed for insurance purposes, they represented "population averages" (not "ideals") based on actuarial data drawn from a large sample of people. For these reasons, nowadays, instead of weight/ height tables, body mass index (BMI) is the gauge used by most fitness experts, nutritionists, medical researchers, and government agencies to determine whether an individual's weight is appropriate for his/her height.

BMI is calculated by dividing the body weight in kilograms by the square of the height in meters. To learn how to calculate your BMI in either metric or standard measurements, see the examples presented below. Alternatively, the table below presents BMIs for different heights and weights. To read the table, find the appropriate height in the left column, and then move across the row to the weight closest to yours. The number at the top is the BMI for that height and weight.

For adults up through middle-age, a BMI between 20 and 27 falls within the desirable range; a BMI over 27 indicates over-

Determining Your Body Mass Index (BMI)

Calculating BMI (in metric measurements)

Determine your height in meters
  (e.g., 165 cm = 1.65 meters)

Square that number
  (1.65 x 1.65 = 2.7225)

Divide your weight in kilograms by the result (65 ÷ 2.7225 = **23.875**)

Calculating BMI (in standard measurements)

Determine your height in inches
  (e.g., 5 feet 5 inches = 65 inches)

Square that number (65 x 65 = 4225)

Divide your weight in pounds by the result
  (e.g., 140 ÷ 4225 = 0.0331)

Multiply that number by 703 (0.0331 x 703 = **23.27**)

Table of body mass indexes—standard measurements

BMI (kg/m2)	19	20	21	22	23	24	25	26	27	28	29	30	35	40
Height (in.)						Body Weight (lbs.)								
58	91	96	100	105	110	115	119	124	129	134	138	143	167	191
59	94	99	104	109	114	119	124	128	133	138	143	148	173	198
60	97	102	107	112	118	123	128	133	138	143	148	153	179	204
61	100	106	111	116	122	127	132	137	143	148	153	158	185	211
62	104	109	115	120	126	131	136	142	147	153	158	164	191	218
63	107	113	118	124	130	135	141	146	152	158	163	169	197	225
64	110	116	122	128	134	140	145	151	157	163	169	174	204	232
65	114	120	126	132	138	144	150	156	162	168	174	180	210	240
66	118	124	130	136	142	148	155	161	167	173	179	186	216	247
67	121	127	134	140	146	153	159	166	172	178	185	191	223	255
68	125	131	138	144	151	158	164	171	177	184	190	197	230	262
69	128	135	142	149	155	162	169	176	182	189	196	203	236	270
70	132	139	146	153	160	167	174	181	188	195	202	207	243	278
71	136	143	150	157	165	172	179	186	193	200	208	215	250	286
72	140	147	154	162	169	177	184	191	199	206	213	221	258	294
73	144	151	159	166	174	182	189	197	204	212	219	227	265	302
74	148	155	163	171	179	186	194	202	210	218	225	233	272	311
75	152	160	168	176	184	192	200	208	216	224	232	240	279	319
76	156	164	172	180	189	197	205	213	221	230	238	246	287	328

(Source: Consumer.gov, a resource sponsored by the U.S. federal government: www.consumer.gov/weightloss/bmi.htm)

weight; and a BMI above 29 indicates obesity. Children and pregnant women have different BMI guidelines. (The World Health Organization's classification of what represents normal, overweight, and obese for the overall adult population is marginally different from the classification provided by the U.S. government: A normal BMI is between 18.5 and 24.9; overweight is between 25 and 29.9; and obese is over 30.)

The BMI is an improvement over weight/height tables because it is based on an individual's body mass rather than on a sample of people, but it still does not provide a measure of the fatness or leanness of the body. To do that, one's body-fat content must be assessed (see next section).

Body Fat

A more accurate guide to ideal weight and "fatness" is to take a direct measurement of body fat. The average fat content of a young, healthy adult male is 10–15 percent and for a young, healthy woman is 18–25 percent. The higher the age, typically the greater the fat content. Therefore an upward adjustment of some 10 percent might be made for older individuals, although from a health perspective such an adjustment may not necessarily be desirable.

While direct measurement has the potential to provide the most accurate assessment of body fat, the technologies available for taking such measurements have limitations. The most common technique is to measure skinfold thickness using calipers in the areas of the biceps, triceps, back (subscapular, or just below the scapula), top of the hip (suprailiac), and thighs. This measure, however, can be inaccurate because skin fold calipers cannot open wide enough to measure total fat thickness in the case of the very obese. Moreover, the measure assumes that 50 percent of body fat is located in subcutaneal tissues, that is, directly beneath the skin. This, however, is not necessarily so, because body form, nutrition, and physical activity can influence how fat is distributed around the body.

Pulse Rate

The resting pulse rate is a good indicator of cardiovascular fitness, because it shows the character and rate at which the heart contracts to pump blood to the lungs and the rest of the body. Pulse rates should be measured under calm conditions, using the pulse that can be felt on the radial artery of the wrist. Alternatively, the pulse that can be felt on the carotid artery, in the neck just below the angle of the jaw, can be used. The pulse is taken for either 6, 10, or 15 seconds and then multiplied by 10, 6, or 4 respectively to derive the beats per minute. The normal resting pulse rate is between 60 and 70 beats per minute.

World Health Organization's Classification of Blood Pressure		
Classification	Systolic (mm/Hg)	Diastolic (mm/Hg)
Low	less than 90	less than 60
Normal	90–139	60–89
High normal/borderline hypertension	140–160	90–95
Above average	above 160	above 95
Note: mm/Hg refers to millimeters (mm) of mercury (Hg)		

Blood Pressure

A person's resting blood pressure indicates the pressure involved when the heart contracts (systolic phase) and relaxes (diastolic phase). Blood pressure outside the normal range indicates poor health and the possibility of cardiovascular illness. A typical blood pressure for a young adult is 120 (systolic) over 70 (diastolic). The risk factor rises with blood pressure rates measuring 140/90 and more; therefore, a rate higher than either of those numbers requires medical clearance prior to exercise (see also Chapter 3, section titled "Cardiac Muscle"). Medical clearance before exercise is also needed in cases of low blood pressure. The World Health Organization's classification of blood pressure is provided above.

Strength

Strength is measured by the force that can be exerted to undertake a physical task. Two measures are commonly used: handgrip strength and sit-ups (abdominal crunches). A handgrip dynamometer is used to measure handgrip strength.

Stamina and Endurance

Stamina is tested using several different measures. Common measures generally include counting the number of abdominal crunches that can be executed and the "step" test. The type of step test used may vary, but basically it requires the individual to step up and down on a step-box with alternating feet at a steady pace for a period of 3 minutes, after which the heart rate is measured and compared against a chart. The lower the heartbeat after executing the steps, the greater the stamina. A heart rate lower than 112 beats per minute for men and lower than 109 beats per minute for women is generally rated excellent. For both men and women, heartbeats exceeding 136 are rated poor. The step test is a convenient and simple measure, but its reliance on the maintenance of regular stepping frequency and variations in people's leg length and weight can all reduce the consistency of the results.

In determining cardiorespiratory endurance or stamina, the most common approach is to measure the oxygen uptake (volume of oxygen inhaled) during exercise on a treadmill, rowing machine, bicycle, or similar appliance used for aerobic activities.

Flexibility

Flexibility tests can measure either static or dynamic flexibility. Static flexibility is determined by the extent muscles and joints can facilitate a movement, while dynamic flexibility refers to the ease of movement. Dynamic flexibility is important for exercises such as gymnastics and dance; static flexibility is important for yoga. Generally, only static flexibility is measured. A sit-and-reach technique is normally used to measure the flexibility of the back and hamstrings (figure A, page 16), two groups of muscles that are generally sources of tightness. The further the reach, the greater the flexibility. A hamstring test (figure B, page 16) provides an alternative method for measuring the flexibility of the hamstrings. In the shoulder test (figure C, page 16), extending the arms behind the ears indicates greater flexibility, but arms held to the front show stiffness in the shoulders. In the quadriceps test (figure D, page 16), the closer the heel to the buttock, the more flexible the thigh.

Ready, Set, Go!

Medical check-ups and fitness testing can seem daunting, but they are usually the prelude to years of safe and enjoyable activity that brings enormous benefits, keeping you mobile, active, and young. Gaining strength, flexibility, endurance, and coordination empowers you to do the things you wish to do, giving you confidence and independence. It means moving better. Posture improves so that you stand taller and reach out farther.

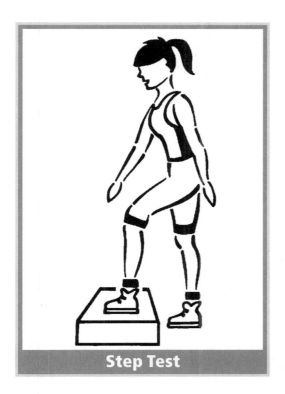

Step Test

The body becomes toned and tauter. Fatigue is reduced and energy levels increase.

These benefits by themselves are sufficient to promote the feel-good factor. There is, however, much, much more to be gained as your muscles, bones, heart, lungs, circulatory system, and body cells change in response to exercise. The efficiency and strength of muscles improve as the number of component muscle fibers rises; weight-bearing activities increase the density of bones, making them stronger and less prone to breakage; joints are more mobile; the heart and lungs become larger and stronger and better equipped to deal with the stress of modern living; and the skin improves with better circulation and respiration. Even the hormonal balance of the body is improved, bringing a tremendous sense of well-being.

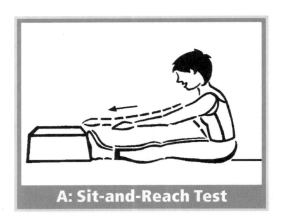

A: Sit-and-Reach Test

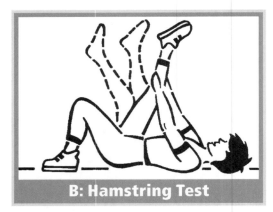

B: Hamstring Test

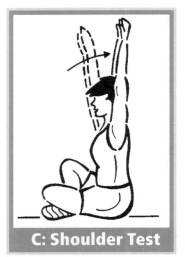

C: Shoulder Test

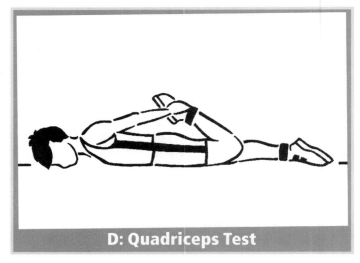

D: Quadriceps Test

Understanding Your Body and Its Responses to Exercise

To understand and maximize the benefits of exercise, it is vital to understand how the body works. Doing so helps to set realistic targets and objectives when setting out to improve performance, body shape, and health.

The Skeleton

The human adult has a total of 213 bones (counting the fused bones in the sacrum [5] and coccyx [4] as individual bones). The bones are joined with ligaments and tendons to form a framework which supports the attached muscles and protects the soft tissues and internal organs. The cranium, for example, protects the brain; the ribs provide similar protection for the heart and lungs, as well as maintaining the chest cavity; the pelvis protects the reproductive organs; and the backbone encloses the spinal cord. This framework determines a person's basic shape.

The bony framework of the body consists of two major parts: the *axial skeleton* (87 bones) consisting of the skull, spine, ribs, and sternum; and the *appendicular skeleton* (126 bones) consisting of two limb girdles—the shoulder and the pelvis—and their attached limb bones.

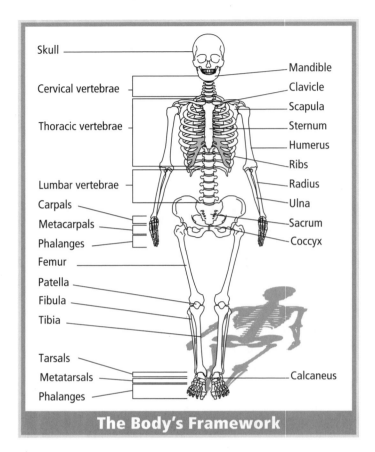

Skull

Cervical vertebrae

Thoracic vertebrae

Lumbar vertebrae

Carpals

Metacarpals

Phalanges

Femur

Patella

Fibula

Tibia

Tarsals

Metatarsals

Phalanges

Mandible

Clavicle

Scapula

Sternum

Humerus

Ribs

Radius

Ulna

Sacrum

Coccyx

Calcaneus

The Body's Framework

The shape and function of bones differ. Long bones, such as the humerus, ulna, and radius in the arm and the femur, fibula, and tibia in the leg, act as levers and are principal movers. Short bones, such as the patella (knee cap), tarsals (located in the foot), and carpals (located in the hands), can engage only in restricted movement. Flat bones, which include the cranium, scapula, sternum, and pelvis, have protective functions. Irregular bones, such as the vertebrae, provide support to the body. The vertebrae also have the vital job of protect-ing the spinal cord: Each vertebra has a central passage through which the spinal cord runs. The spinal cord is a cylinder of nerve tissues and can be represented as a downward extension of the brain. Together, the brain and the spinal cord form the cen-tral nervous system, which is responsible for, among other vital functions, the control of body movements.

Bones and Their Development

Bones are not inert; they provide a mobile framework on which muscles act to produce

The Spinal Column

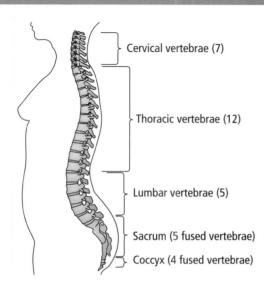

Cervical vertebrae (7)

Thoracic vertebrae (12)

Lumbar vertebrae (5)

Sacrum (5 fused vertebrae)

Coccyx (4 fused vertebrae)

The human spine consists of thirty-three vertebrae grouped in three sections: the cervical vertebrae, which support the head and neck; the thoracic vertebrae, to which the ribs are attached; and the lower back, consisting of the lumbar, the sacrum, and the coccyx. Together, the lumbar, sacrum, and coccyx form a stable center for the body during movement.

The vertebrae are connected by facet joints, which provide stability to the spine yet allow movement. Between the vertebrae are the intervertebral discs, tough, fibrous, cartilage discs that help cushion the force of the body's movements. Injury to these discs results in pressure on the spinal nerves, which in turn causes pain. The vertebrae are held together by ligaments. Bony protrusions from the vertebrae provide sites for the attachment of muscles. The spinal cord, a network of nerve tissues, runs within the spinal column. Spinal nerves pass from the spinal cord to the body through gaps between the vertebrae.

Normally, the spine curves gently forward in the cervical region, slightly backward in the thoracic region, and slightly forward in the lumbar region. The spinal structure limits the ability of the body to bend backwards, but allows it to bend forward easily. When this natural curvature is unbalanced, as a result of poor posture, weak abdominal muscles, congenital defects, or bone diseases, back disorders result; these are often extremely painful. Lordosis, excessive inward curvature of the lower back, and kyphosis, excessive rearward curvature of the upper spine, are both associated with poor posture, excess weight, and weak abdominal muscles.

Correct body alignment is essential in our daily activities and in exercise if spinal disorders are to be avoided. Back pain is one of the most common afflictions of modern society and affects almost everyone sometime during the course of their lives. You will find in the chapters on exercises that special emphasis is placed on maintaining correct alignment of the spine, particularly the lower back.

movements. The inner core of the bones, the bone marrow, is the site of production of both red and white blood cells. Bones also store minerals, particularly calcium and phosphorus, that other parts of the body can draw upon when needed. The stronger the bones, the greater the strength of the skeleton. Exercise can contribute significantly to bone strength.

The development of the skeleton is a lengthy process that starts in the womb and is only completed in early adulthood. Most bones begin to develop in the human embryo in the fifth or sixth week of pregnancy. By about seven weeks, the embryo will have the rudiments of most of the bones of the body, but at this early stage they are soft and flexible. Most of these structures are made of cartilage, but a few are only membranes. For example, some of the facial bones, most of the brain case, and the collarbones start as membranes in the embryo. Around the eighth week, bone begins to form in the cartilage and membranes through the process of ossification. Special cells, called *osteoblasts*, move out from the center of the cartilage and membranes, depositing calcium carbonate and calcium phosphate, the main ingredients of bone.

By the time a baby is born, much of the ossification is complete, but the bones are by no means completely formed. For example, a conspicuous soft spot, the fontanel, exists at the top of a newborn baby's head for several months. If the skull bone were not flexible, babies would be unable to pass through the opening in their mother's pelvic girdle.

The formation of bone can be likened to a battle between the osteoblasts, which encourage the deposition of the bone minerals, and the *osteoclasts*, which remove mineral from the bone. Bone is continuously being made and resorbed in response to secretions of various hormones, including growth hormones, the sex hormones (estrogen and testosterone), adrenal hormones, and parathyroid and thyroid hormones. These hormones control the amount of calcium in the blood.

During the growth period, bone density increases, making the bone hard and resilient as a result of hormonal stimulation of the osteoblasts. Because the bones are rigid, they grow in specific areas that remain active after the rest of the bone has become completely ossified. The long limb bones, for example, have a growth disk near each end (the epiphyses) that enables the bone to lengthen during childhood growth. After adolescence, the growth disks also become ossified and bone growth ceases. Some parts of the skeleton, such as the external ears, the tip of the nose, and the ends of bones where they meet to form a joint, remain as cartilage.

People start to lose bone density in their mid-thirties. This loss of bone, known as *osteoporosis*, is a natural part of aging. In contrast to the growth period, in osteoporosis the osteoclasts appear to have the upper hand. By the age of 70 the male skeleton will have lost on average about 10 percent of its bone, while the bone in the female skeleton will have been reduced by about 25 percent. The process is particularly fast in women after menopause because of the loss of estrogen. The reduction in bone density increases the brittleness of bones and their vulnerability to fracture. By the age of 75 about half of all women will have suffered a fracture as a result of osteoporosis.

The decrease in bone density can be slowed down by regular weight-bearing exercises such as walking, jogging, aerobics, ice skating, skipping, and dancing. These activities encourage bone formation by involving the skeletal framework in bearing the body's weight, in contrast to activities such as swimming and aqua-aerobics, in which the body's weight is offset by its buoyancy in water. The earlier in life an individual commences weight-bearing activities, the stronger the bones are likely to be. In addition, the *periosteum*, the thin membrane that covers the bone and contains a network of blood and nerve vessels, also benefits from the increased blood supply that results from regular physical activity.

Joints

A *joint* is the junction between two or more bones. Joints, together with bones and muscles, feature very importantly in determining the type of movements that can be produced. Bones are joined together by *ligaments*, which are tough fibrous tissues that give joints stability. Ligaments are relatively inelastic and have a limited response to sudden movements at the joint. Sudden excessive movements can result in damage, and a torn ligament can take at least 6 months and sometimes even years to repair. In some instances the damage may be permanent, because ligaments have a poor blood supply and as a result do not repair easily. Another fibrous cord, the *tendon*, is also involved in movement. Tendons consist of bundles of collagen (white fibrous protein); they join bone to muscle or muscle to muscle. They are strong and flexible, but inelastic. They can also be damaged by excessive sudden movements, but because they have a blood supply they heal faster than ligaments.

Some joints, such as those in the skull, are fixed, because the bones are fused or held together by collagen. Some joints allow only restricted movement; they are called *partially movable joints*. Included in this category are the ellipsoidal joints such as the wrist and ankle. They allow movement from side to side and up and down. Pivot joints allow only rotational movements. An example is the joint between the first cervical vertebra at the base of the skull, which rotates around the second cervical vertebra. *Mobile*, or *movable*, *joints* include hinge joints and ball-and-socket joints. Hinge joints, such as those in the elbows, knees, fingers, and toes, allow bending and straightening. The elbow and knee also

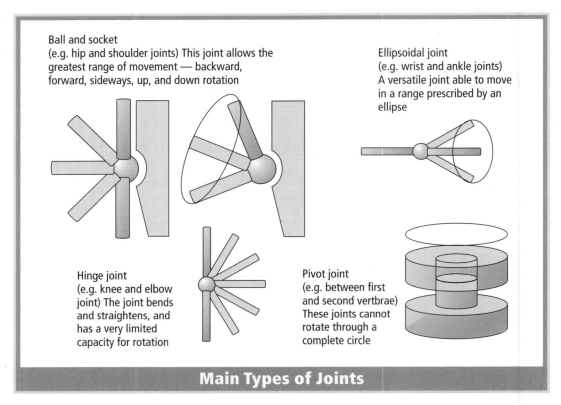

Ball and socket
(e.g. hip and shoulder joints) This joint allows the greatest range of movement — backward, forward, sideways, up, and down rotation

Ellipsoidal joint
(e.g. wrist and ankle joints) A versatile joint able to move in a range prescribed by an ellipse

Hinge joint
(e.g. knee and elbow joint) The joint bends and straightens, and has a very limited capacity for rotation

Pivot joint
(e.g. between first and second vertbrae) These joints cannot rotate through a complete circle

Main Types of Joints

provide for limited rotation. Ball-and-socket joints allow the widest range of movements in all directions, including backward, forward, sideways, and rotation (see illustration above). Examples are the shoulder and the hip.

To facilitate movements, partially movable and movable joints are specially structured. The bone surface is coated with smooth cartilage to reduce friction and act as a shock absorber. The joint is enclosed by the *joint capsule*. This tough fibrous capsule is lined by the *synovial membrane*, which produces a sticky fluid that acts as a

lubricant where the bones meet. Each joint is surrounded by strong ligaments that support the joint, provide stability, and prevent excessive movement. Movements are produced and controlled by muscles attached to the bone, usually via a tendon.

It is important in any exercise regime to warm up with mobilizing movements that concentrate on the joints. The warming-up process brings heat to the thick synovial fluid. Thinning of the synovial fluid helps to cushion impact and friction; this "oiling" effect also helps to increase the range of

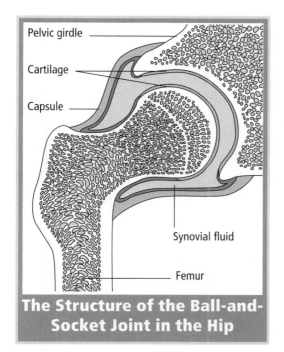

Pelvic girdle

Cartilage

Capsule

Synovial fluid

Femur

The Structure of the Ball-and-Socket Joint in the Hip

movements, preparing the ligaments and tendons for more strenuous activity.

The Muscles

Muscles consist of bundles of specialized cells that are capable of contracting and relaxing to create movement of the body or of organs within it. Three types of muscles exist in the body: *skeletal* or *striated muscle*, *smooth muscle*, and *cardiac muscle*. Skeletal muscle is sometimes called *voluntary muscle*, because apart from reflex actions it is subject to conscious control by the brain. Smooth muscle is often called *involuntary muscle* because it is not controlled con-

sciously but rather responds to hormonal and involuntary nervous stimuli.

Skeletal Muscle
How the Skeletal Muscles Work
Skeletal muscles, as the name suggests, are linked to the skeleton of the body. There are some 600 of them, and they are classified by the movements that they produce. The point where a muscle is attached to the more stable bone is generally referred to as the *point of origin* or *attachment*, while the point where the muscle connects with the movable bone is commonly referred to as the *point of insertion*.

An *extensor muscle* extends or opens a joint. A good example is the *triceps*, a muscle situated at the back of the arm. It has three heads (hence its name) attached to corresponding points of origin, one in the *scapula* and two in the upper part of the *humerus*. The lower end of the triceps is attached to a large tendon that inserts into the *ulna* bone below the elbow joint. When the triceps contracts, the forearm straightens or extends.

A *flexor muscle* closes the joint. Keeping to the example of the arm, the *biceps* is a flexor muscle. This muscle has two points of origin, at the tip of the *coracoid process* in the scapula and the top of the scapula, respectively, and inserts into the *radius*. When the biceps contracts, the elbow

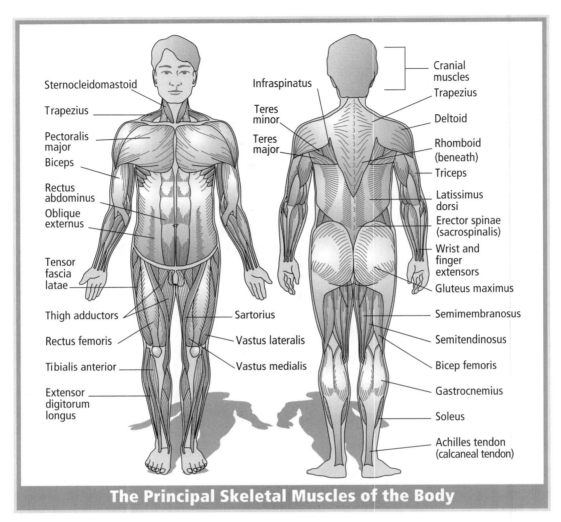

The Principal Skeletal Muscles of the Body

bends, bringing the forearm inward. Its contraction can also rotate the forearm.

Muscles responsible for moving a bone outward are classified as *abductors*, and those that bring them inward are called *adductors*. The *deltoid*, the triangular muscle in the outer upper arm, and the muscles in the upper outer part of the thigh, the *tensor fascia latae*, are abductors. When they contract, they move the arm and leg respectively outward. The muscles in the upper inner thigh, the *adductor brevis*, *adductor longus*, and *adductor magnus*, move the leg inward. Other adductor muscles include the *pectorals*, the chest muscles originating from the *sternum* and *clavicle* and inserting into the *humerus*, and the *teres major* and *teres minor*, originating from the edge of the scapula and inserting into the back of the humerus just below the shoulder. These work in conjunction with the *latissimus dorsi*, running from the *spine* to the *humerus* to move the arm inward.

Other categories of muscles include *levators* and *depressors*, responsible, respectively, for raising and lowering, and *sphincter muscles*, for constriction. See the table titled "The Skeletal Muscles of the Body" on pages 27–30 for basic information on the major muscle groups.

From the descriptions given you can see that individual muscles do not work alone. When the biceps contracts to move the forearm inward, it cannot then straighten on its own but will do so when the triceps, the *opposing* or *antagonist* muscle, contracts to extend the forearm. Thus, muscles lengthen via the action of the opposing muscle group. Movement is produced only when a muscle crosses a joint, in this case the elbow. A muscle may cross a number of joints before it reaches the site of its principal action. In order to prevent unwanted movements in the other joints, groups of muscles known as *synergist muscles* contract to stabilize them.

Muscles rely on contraction to produce movements. In other words, they pull, but they cannot push. In any single action there will be a muscle that is the prime mover (*agonist*), an opposing (*antagonist*) muscle that relaxes to support this move, and *synergist*

muscles (in the intermediate joints) that stabilize the action around the joints. Thus, in bending the forearm inward, the biceps is the prime mover or agonist and the triceps is the antagonist, while in straightening the arm, the triceps is the prime mover and the biceps the antagonist (see figure on page 26).

Understanding the points of origin, points of insertion, and the joints/bones involved when contracting a muscle is essential for an instructor who wants to tailor specific exercises for specific muscle groups. Not only does such knowledge help to target the muscles to be worked, it helps to reduce the strain that can occur from improper positioning of the body. The latter is often a result of inadequate understanding of the principles of muscle contraction, insertion, and origin.

For example, full sit-ups and "stomach crunches" (raising the trunk by about 30 degrees) are performed to strengthen the stomach muscles, the *rectus abdominus*. If these movements are made with the legs extended straight out on the floor, there will be stress and strain on the lower back, because the *hip flexor/iliopsoas* muscle acts synergistically, contracting to stabilize the hip and allowing the trunk to be raised. In doing so, it pulls the lower back and causes stress in the lumbar region. This stress can be avoided, however, if the exercise is performed with the legs bent. Bending the legs

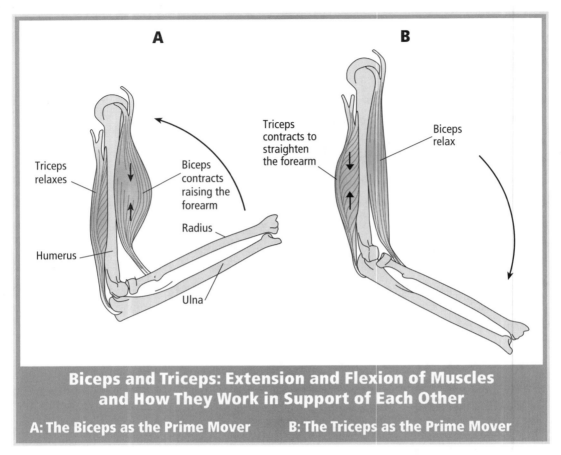

A

B

Triceps relaxes

Biceps contracts raising the forearm

Radius

Humerus

Ulna

Triceps contracts to straighten the forearm

Biceps relax

Biceps and Triceps: Extension and Flexion of Muscles and How They Work in Support of Each Other

A: The Biceps as the Prime Mover   **B: The Triceps as the Prime Mover**

involves the iliopsoas and will stabilize the hip area *before* starting the trunk movement, thereby avoiding the stress in the back that occurs when the muscles act simultaneously in an opposite direction. Even better would be to contract the *transverse abdominal* muscles as well, which would provide greater stability in the lower trunk and focus the exercise on the rectus abdominus. (A detailed, step-by-step description of this exercise is given on pages 92–93 and page 104.)

The principles governing the actions of muscles and the resulting body movements form the cornerstone of aerobic routines and fitness training. In brief, these movements are

- flexion (e.g., bending the arm or leg)

- extension (e.g., straightening the arm or leg)

- abduction (e.g., lifting the arm or leg sideways away from the body)

- adduction (e.g., crossing the leg)

The Skeletal Muscles of the Body

Muscle	Origin	Insertion	Joints crossed	Movement
UPPER BODY				
Sternocleidomastoid	Top of sternum and inner end of clavicle	Skull, mastoid process at back of head, and behind ears	Neck	Flexes head, drawing it towards shoulder; rotation of head
Biceps	Scapula	Radius	Shoulder/elbow	Flexion of forearm; supination of forearm, i.e., turning palm upwards
Triceps	Top and rear of humerus and edge of scapula	Ulna	Shoulder/elbow	Straightens forearm; extension of shoulder
Deltoids	Clavicle and scapula	Humerus	Shoulder	Abducts or lifts shoulder away from the body, i.e., extends and flexes upper arm
Pectoralis major	Clavicle and sternum	Humerus	Shoulder	Adduction of humerus, i.e., moves upper arm inward across the body
Rectus abdominus	Pubis	Middle ribs (5th, 6th, and 7th)	Pelvis and trunk	Pelvic tilt, trunk flexion
Transverse abdominus	Thoracic lumbar region of the spine (between iliac crest and 12th rib)	Pubis via internal obliques and rectus abdominus	Pelvis and trunk	Constricts and supports the abdomen and helps force air out of the lungs
External obliques	Eight lower ribs	Iliac crest	Pelvis and trunk	Flexes, rotates, and bends trunk

The Skeletal Muscles of the Body (cont'd.)

Muscle	Origin	Insertion	Joints crossed	Movement
UPPER BODY				
Internal obliques	Iliac crest	7th to 9th costal (rib) cartilages; lower fibers join the aponeurosis of the transverse abdominus and insert in the pubic crest	Pelvis and trunk	Flexes, rotates, and side bends trunk
Erector spinae	Sacrum, ilium, lower spinous processes of the lumbar, lower ribs	Spinous processes stretching from 1st cervical to 5th lumbar	Trunk	Extension of back; lateral flexion, rotation of the vertebral column; lateral movement of the pelvis
Transversospinalis-multifidus	Laminae of vertebrae	Spinous processes 2 or 3 vertebrae above	Trunk	Lateral flexion, rotation, extension/hyperextension of spine
Rhomboids	Spinous processes from 7th cervical and upper 5 thoracic vertebrae	Inner part of the scapula	Juncture of scapula, spine, and upper ribs	Adduction of scapula towards spine
Trapezius	Spinous processes from the base of skull (7th cervical vertebra), along the 1st–5th thoracic vertebrae, down to the 6th–12th thoracic vertebrae	Clavicle and upper and middle scapula	Juncture of scapula, spine, upper ribs, and shoulder	Adducts, rotates, and elevates scapula; laterally flexes neck

The Skeletal Muscles of the Body (cont'd.)

Muscle	Origin	Insertion	Joints crossed	Movement
UPPER BODY				
Latissimus dorsi	Spinous processes stretching from 6 lower thoracic vertebrae to 5 lumbar vertebrae and the posterior crest of the ilium (pelvis)	Humerus	Shoulder	Pulls arm downward and backward and rotates humerus medially, i.e., draws arm back and inward towards the body
LOWER BODY				
Iliopsoas/ hip flexor	Stretching from front of 12th thoracic vertebra to 5th lumbar vertebra and front of ilium	Top inside of femur	Hip/pelvic joint	Flexes hip; lateral rotation of femur
Quadriceps: rectus femoris	Front of ilium	Patella and tibia	Hip/pelvic joint and knee	Extension of knee, leg; flexion of thigh at hip
Abductors: tensor fascia latae	Outer edge and front of ilium	Top, outer part of tibia	Hip/knee	Flexion, abduction, and medial rotation of thigh
Tibialis anterior	Front, outer side of tibia, just below knee	Inner edge of foot, before big toe	Ankle	Dorsi flexion, i.e., flexing foot upwards
Gluteals: gluteus maximus	Back of ilium and along sacroiliac joint	Top of femur	Hip/pelvic joint	Extension of thigh (lifting leg backward); lateral rotation of leg

The Skeletal Muscles of the Body (cont'd.)				
Muscle	Origin	Insertion	Joints crossed	Movement
LOWER BODY				
Hamstring	Ischium	Tibia	Knee	Flexes knee; extension of thigh
Adductors: adductus brevis, longus, magnus	Front part of pubic bone and lower hip bone	Femur stretching from hip to knee	Hip	Adduction of leg; hip flexion; lateral rotation of thigh
Gastrocnemius	Back of femur, just above knee	Achilles calcaneous/heel bone	Knee/ankle	Knee flexion; plantar flexion (pointing of toes)
Soleus	Outside and back of tibia, just below knee	Achilles calcaneous/ heel bone	Ankle	Plantar flexion (pointing of toes)

- circumduction (e.g., circling the arm)

- pronation (e.g., turning the foot or hand inward)

- supination (e.g., turning the foot or hand outward)

- plantar flexion (e.g., pointing the toes downward)

- dorsi flexion (e.g., flexing the foot to point the toes upward)

These terms may seem rather technical, but anyone who has been to an aerobic class would easily recognize them in typical movements such as "biceps curls" or "hamstring curls" (flexion) or "windmill arms"

(circumduction). The step known as "grapevine" involves abduction, that is, moving one leg to the side, and adduction, bringing the other leg inward. "Squats" involve flexion of the thigh. "Heel digs" involve dorsi flexion, and so on.

How the Muscle Fibers Work
Skeletal muscles consist of bundles of muscle fibers composed of elongated cells enclosed in a tough sheath of tissue. Each end of a muscle is drawn out to form tendons that are attached to the tough membrane, the periosteum, that surrounds the bones of the skeleton. Muscles vary in size according to the number of bundles that they contain.

A large muscle such as the gluteus maximus (the large powerful muscle in the buttocks) or the rectus femoris (the largest muscle in the quadriceps) contains thousands of bundles of muscle fibers. A small muscle such as the triceps contains far fewer bundles.

Each muscle fiber consists of smaller fibers or *myofibrils*, which contain alternating thick and thin microscopic filaments. The thick filament mostly consists of the protein *myosin*, while the thin filament mostly consists of the protein *actin*. The alignment of the thick and thin filaments in bands accounts for the typical striated or striped appearance of these muscle fibers when viewed with a microscope. As a result, skeletal muscle is often referred to as *striated muscle*. The functional unit of these protein filaments that is responsible for muscular contraction is called a *sarcomere*.

Muscle contraction is produced when the brain sends out a signal that is relayed to the muscle fiber via nerve endings. The nerve impulse stimulates the muscle by releasing chemicals from the nerve endings. This starts a chain of reactions that results in the myosin and actin filaments sliding over each other in an action akin to the closing of an extendable ladder, with the filaments hooking on to each other. This shortens the sarcomere, and so the muscle fibers contract.

The bigger the muscle the greater its strength, because of the larger number of fibers that can be brought into use. Lifting a small object requires the use of far fewer muscle fibers than when lifting large objects. Hence, if you were to lift a small potted plant, the number of muscle fibers you recruit would be much smaller than if you were to lift a big potted plant. This recruitment of muscle fibers can be learned and modified through experience.

Most of us are totally unaware of the brain, eye, and muscle coordination that is

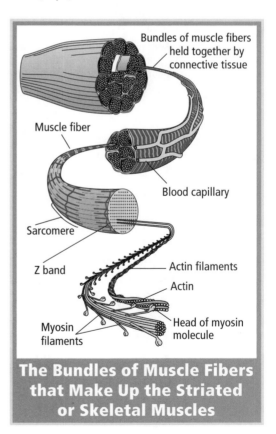

Bundles of muscle fibers held together by connective tissue

Muscle fiber

Blood capillary

Sarcomere

Z band

Actin filaments

Actin

Myosin filaments

Head of myosin molecule

The Bundles of Muscle Fibers that Make Up the Striated or Skeletal Muscles

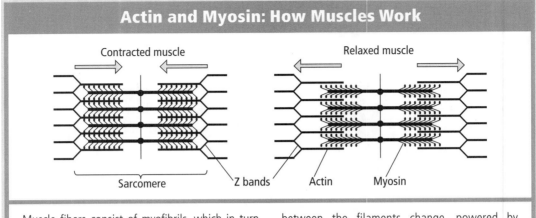

Actin and Myosin: How Muscles Work

Contracted muscle

Relaxed muscle

Sarcomere   Z bands   Actin   Myosin

Muscle fibers consist of myofibrils, which in turn are made up of two myofilaments, a thin one consisting mainly of the protein actin, and a thicker one made up mainly of the protein myosin. During muscle contraction, hooklike attachments between the filaments change, powered by chemical energy, sliding them together. The boundary between each contractile unit, known as a sarcomere, is called the Z-band; it provides an anchorage for the myofilaments

involved routinely in controlling our movements and posture. It can be very startling, therefore, if for some reason the strength required to move an object is wrongly judged. This can be demonstrated by a very simple experiment. Find two identical cans with lids; leave one empty and fill the other with sand. Put them on a table; ask an unsuspecting friend to pass you the filled can, and then ask immediately afterward for the empty one. The recruitment of muscle fibers necessary to lift the first, heavy can will have been registered in the brain. Invariably, with no contradictory visual or other clues, the same force will be applied to the empty, light can. As a result the hand and can will move quickly and involuntarily upward before the brain can correct its error.

Such is the "shock" of this failure in coordination that it is difficult to repeat the experiment with the same individual or someone who has seen it done, even if the identical cans are rearranged while the person's back is turned. The next time you ask the person to pass the cans, he will assess the weight of each one before lifting them. Of course, some experiences are deepseated and require an effort to readjust from, as anyone who has walked down a stationary escalator or come ashore after a long sailing trip will know.

We are able to control and modify the actions of skeletal muscles because structures called *proprioceptors* provide feedback on the physical movement and changes in tension or force to the brain, which can then send the appropriate stimuli to the muscles (see diagram below on the Motor Nervous System). Essentially, there are three kinds of proprioceptors, although they can be subdivided according to form and specific function:

- *neuromuscular* or *muscle spindles*, which are embedded in the muscles

- *Golgi tendon organs*, which lie close to where the muscle sheath attaches to the tendon

- *joint receptors*, situated mainly in and near the articular capsules of joints, close to the Golgi tendon organs

The muscle spindles, which lie parallel to the muscle fibers, provide feedback on the length of the muscle, and during movement they monitor the degree and speed with which it is being stretched. If the muscle is being overstretched, the spindles signal the need to contract the muscle. The Golgi tendon organs monitor the force exerted on the tendons by the muscle at rest, but they become particularly active when it contracts. In contrast to the muscle spindles, they signal the need for the muscle to relax in order to reduce the force being exerted. Both proprioceptors work together, the spindles regulating muscular tension to

produce a smooth movement and the tendon organs regulating the force applied by the muscles to prevent injury and damage to the muscles, tendons, and bones. The picture is completed by the joint receptors, which provide information on the angle of joints, the pressure exerted on them, and, when moving, acceleration.

In the case of the can experiment, it is easy to imagine how all these elements combine with other sensory information to supply the brain with the information necessary to coordinate movement and correct

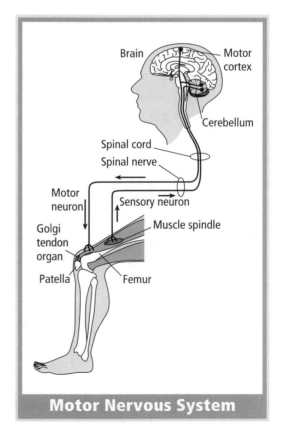

Motor Nervous System

its mistake. Being aware of the proprioceptors is important when exercising. Most importantly, you should be guided by messages delivered by the tendon organs and avoid overriding their messages, for example by trying to lift excessively heavy weights or attempting to exert excessive force when using equipment. On the other hand, to stretch adequately at the end of a workout, you must hold the stretch for at least 25 to 30 seconds beyond the point when the muscle first tightens as a result of the response of the muscle spindles.

Fast- and Slow-Twitch Muscle Fibers

Skeletal muscles consist of two different kinds of muscle fiber, *fast-twitch* and *slow-twitch* fibers, the preponderance of which determines both the appearance and capacities of muscles. Fast-twitch muscles are white and respond very quickly to stimulation. They have a better capacity for anaerobic metabolism, which means they do not need oxygen to power them (see "Energy and Energy Systems" later in this chapter). In contrast, slow-twitch muscle fibers are red in color and have a slower contraction rate. They depend entirely on energy generated by aerobic activities (oxygen) and are red because of their reliance on oxygenated blood supply for energy.

Sports such as sprinting make use of fast-twitch muscles, as do those requiring quick changes of pace, including football, rugby, and basketball. Strength-training activities, which tend to employ anaerobic energy, also use predominantly fast-twitch muscles. In contrast, endurance sports such as marathon and long-distance running use predominantly slow-twitch muscles.

All muscles contain red and white muscle fibers. A cross section of a muscle would illustrate this. But the preponderance of red versus white muscle fibers differs from one part of the body to another and from person to person. A sprinter, for example, would have a very small proportion of slow-twitch muscles compared to a middle- or long-distance runner. A sprinter might have as much as 70 percent of muscle fibers in the fast-twitch form, whereas a long-distance runner might have only 20 percent in this form. An analogy can be made with respect to the color of the breast meat of a domestic chicken and a wild pigeon. A chicken uses its wings to take off suddenly in order to avoid being caught, not for flying as such. Hence the breast muscle, which powers the wings, is predominantly white with fast-twitch fibers for a quick response. A pigeon, however, uses its wings to fly long distances, so the breast muscle is red with predominantly slow-twitch muscle fibers for endurance. Muscles within the chicken itself vary. In contrast to the white muscle fibers of the breast, the leg muscles are much darker because the bird spends most of its time running around on the ground.

This division of the muscle fibers has become blurred, however, in light of recent research showing that training can change the characteristics of muscles. Fast-twitch muscle, which relies primarily on anaerobic energy conversion, can be trained to acquire the slow-twitch characteristic of aerobic respiration. Some evidence also exists that slow-twitch muscles can be converted to fast-twitch if, for example, a marathon runner is trained to sprint. This discovery is important because it shows that training can help to improve both strength and endurance.

The basic structure of the muscle, however, remains all important in shaping athletic and related capacities, and largely determines how individuals respond to training regimes. For example, fast-twitch muscles gain more bulk in response to resistance training, although the situation for women is a little different because they lack sufficient levels of the hormone testosterone. Even so, the predominance of one or the other muscle fiber does influence the results of resistance training. Increased strength in women does not necessarily mean muscle bulk, but increasing the intensity and duration of training can lead to greater muscle definition than usual.

Smooth Muscle

Smooth muscle is responsible for movements in internal organs, such as the uterus, intestines, lungs, bladder, and blood vessels. Smooth muscle does not contain myofibrils. It has thick myosin filaments and thin actin filaments, but these are distributed throughout the muscle cell. Also, smooth muscle has only half the myosin found in skeletal muscle and does not have the sarcomere structure of skeletal muscle. As a result, smooth muscle does not have a striated appearance. Its contraction speed is very slow. Because smooth muscles are not under conscious control, they cannot be trained, but their efficiency and function can be improved indirectly through exercise, especially those geared toward improving the function of the cardiovascular respiratory system.

Cardiac Muscle

The cardiac muscle, or *myocardium*, makes up much of the heart. It contracts rhythmically to propel blood through the circulatory system. It does not need nervous stimulation to contract; isolated cardiac muscle cells, for example, will continue to contract for many hours providing they are bathed in oxygen-rich, nutritious saline. Contraction of the heart is influenced, however, by the involuntary nervous system, hormones, and the stretching of the muscles. Contractions start in the right atrium of the heart, spreading through both atria and then both ventricles alternately.

The Heart and Circulatory System

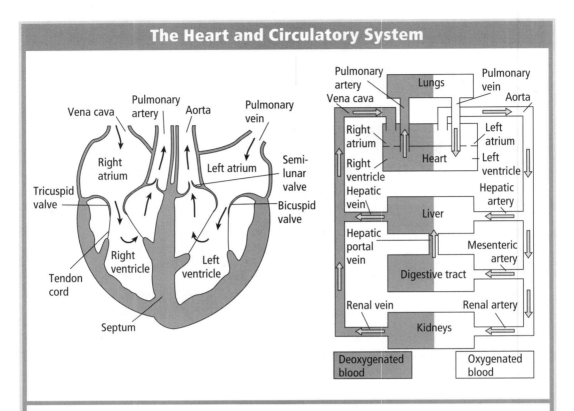

The heart is divided into four chambers: the upper two are called *atria* and the lower two are *ventricles*. The *septum*, which is a thick muscular wall, runs in the center to separate the left atrium and ventricle from the right atrium and ventricle.

The right atrium receives deoxygenated blood from the body via the *vena cava* vein. The buildup of pressure in the right atrium as a result of the inflow pushes the *tricuspid valve* open; this allows deoxygenated blood to be pumped into the right ventricle. The right ventricle contracts to push the blood into the *pulmonary artery*, which leads to the lungs.

In the lungs, the carbon dioxide carried in the blood diffuses into the air sacs *(alveoli)* and is subsequently exhaled, while the oxygen in the alveoli diffuses into the blood. The oxygenated blood is then carried by the *pulmonary vein* to the left atrium of the heart. The *bicuspid valve*, separating the left atrium from the left ventricle, opens, allowing the oxygenated blood to pass into the left ventricle, which then contracts, sending the blood into the *aorta* and out of the heart.

From there, the arterial system distributes the blood throughout the body. The oxygen from the blood is diffused through the capillary walls into the spaces between the body cells. Carbon dioxide passes from body cells via tissue fluids to the capillaries of the venous system, returning eventually to the heart via the vena cava.

The pumping action of the heart varies considerably in response to the demands of the bodily muscles for oxygen. At rest, the heart contracts at around 60 to 70 beats per minute and pushes out some 80 milliliters (ml) of blood at each stroke. During exercise, when more oxygen is needed, the heart can contract at a maximum of 200 to 220 beats per minute to pump over three times the amount of blood it normally pumps. The maximum number of contractions generally reduces with age.

Increases in the heartbeat or myocardial contractions occur during exercise because the active muscles not only require more blood/oxygen, but are also returning more blood. The more blood returning to the heart, the more forcibly the heart can contract to push the blood to the lungs and back around the body. An increase in the contractions of the myocardium contributes to an increase in the strength and size of the heart, just as exercise helps to strengthen skeletal muscles.

Over time, exercise causes advantageous changes to the cardiovascular system. The demands for more blood during exercise lead to an increase in the number of blood capillaries, which helps lower blood pressure. The importance of this is self-evident at a time when the incidence of hypertension (abnormally high blood pressure when at rest) is rising dramatically in the industrialized countries (see sidebar titled "The Cardiac Cycle and Hypertension" on the next page). As the heart becomes stronger, the volume of blood it pushes out at each contraction (*stroke volume*) increases while the resting pulse rate falls. Both changes lower the workload of the heart, reducing the stress and strain.

The Respiratory System

The efficient delivery of oxygen is of paramount importance to the body and brain. This is the job of the pulmonary, or respiratory, system. Air enters through the nose and mouth and passes down the windpipe, or *trachea*. This divides into two *bronchi*, which lead to the left and right lungs, positioned on either side of the heart. Inside the spongy lung the bronchi subdivide into smaller airways called *bronchioles*. Each lung houses some 30,000 of these tiny bronchioles. Each bronchiole divides into two or more respiratory bronchioles, which lead into numerous tiny air sacs, the *alveoli*. Oxygen passes through the thin walls of the alveoli into the bloodstream, and carbon dioxide (the waste product of respiration) passes from the blood into the alveoli to be exhaled.

Each lung is cone-shaped, with the base resting on the *diaphragm*, a sheet of muscle that separates the airtight chest cavity from the abdominal cavity. The right lung is divided into three lobes, and the smaller left

The Cardiac Cycle and Hypertension

The cardiac cycle has three phases: the diastolic, atrial systolic, and ventricle systolic. Together, they make up one heartbeat.

The *diastolic phase* is the resting phase, during which deoxygenated blood flows into the right atrium and oxygenated blood flows into the left atrium. As the blood flows into the atria, the buildup of pressure causes the valves that separate the atria from the ventricles to open so that blood flows simultaneously into the ventricles. About 80 percent of the ventricle is filled with blood at the diastolic phase.

In the *atrial systolic phase*, the atria (both left and right) contract to push more blood into the ventricles to fill them completely. The ventricles then contract, a step referred to as the *ventricle systolic phase*, and the valves that separate the atria from the ventricles close to prevent any flow back. The contraction of the ventricles sends blood out into the arteries—from the right ventricle to the pul-monary artery and from the left ventricle to the aorta.

The amount of blood ejected into the arteries by this contraction is called the *stroke volume*. The amount of blood pushed out per minute is referred to as the *cardiac output*, which is simply stroke volume multiplied by the number of heartbeats that occur during the minute.

Blood pressure generally refers to the pressure exerted on the arteries in the different phases of the cardiac cycle. Blood pressure increases with activity. This is normal. *Hypertension* is when the pressure remains high even at rest.

Blood pressure is measured in two values: the systolic rate and the diastolic rate, or the pressure exerted on the arteries when the ventricles contract, and the pressure exerted during the resting phase. These numbers are expressed in a blood-pressure reading as systolic over diastolic. Normal blood pressure is not strictly defined and varies with age. As people grow older, their body's resistance to blood flow rises because the blood vessels become more rigid, and so blood pressure increases. Generally, blood pressure is normal if it is below 140/90. Individuals with a systolic rate between 140 and 160 and a diastolic rate between 90 and 95 have moderate hypertension. Those with rates exceeding these are classified as having severe hypertension.

It is estimated that between 10 and 20 percent of the adult population in many countries, including the U.K. and the U.S., have hypertension. Men are more prone to it than premenopausal women, but after menopause women become equally susceptible.

Hypertension exists in two forms:

- *primary* or *essential hypertension*, which is without obvious cause, but is linked to gender, lifestyle (smoking, obesity, alcohol), and/or hereditary factors

- *secondary hypertension*, which is linked to specific causes, including kidney disorders, congenital heart defects, and taking certain drugs

Hypertension often passes undetected because there are few obvious symptoms. This is why it is sometimes called the silent killer. Despite the lack of symptoms, hypertension severely increases the stress and strain on the heart, making it susceptible to myocardial infarction (heart attack), stroke, and other coronary heart diseases.

Research studies have proven that regular exercise helps lower blood pressure in all persons suffering from hypertension and therefore protects against heart diseases.

lung is divided into two lobes. Together the lungs form one of the body's largest organs. They provide an internal surface area for the exchange of respiratory gases that is some 40 times greater than the body's outer surface. A *pleural membrane* covers the lungs and lines the thoracic cavity. The membrane produces *pleural fluid*, which lubricates the surfaces of the lungs and tho-racic cavity so that they move easily against one another during breathing.

Air is inhaled and exhaled by the action of the chest muscles (*intercostal* muscles, i.e., between the ribs) and the *diaphragm*. When we inhale, the external intercostal muscles contract, causing the ribs to move upwards and outward, and the diaphragm contracts and flattens, pushing down on the

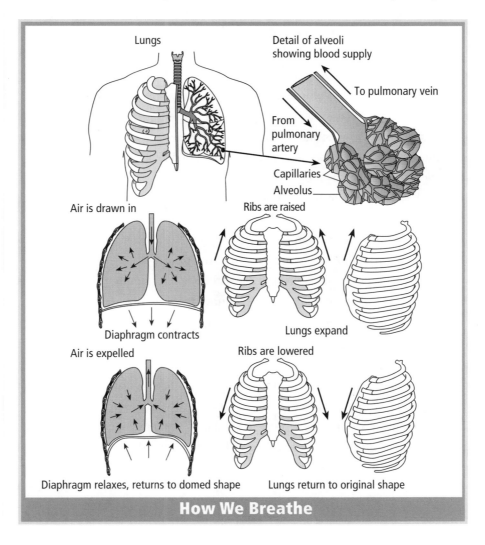

Lungs

Detail of alveoli showing blood supply

To pulmonary vein

From pulmonary artery

Capillaries

Alveolus

Air is drawn in

Diaphragm contracts

Ribs are raised

Lungs expand

Air is expelled

Diaphragm relaxes, returns to domed shape

Ribs are lowered

Lungs return to original shape

How We Breathe

viscera (guts), which are allowed to descend by relaxation of the abdominal wall. This increases the volume of the *thorax* (chest cavity) and of the lungs. The increase in volume raises the capacity of the lungs, so that atmospheric pressure forces air into them. When we exhale, the external intercostal muscles relax and the internal intercostal muscles contract, pushing the ribs downward and inward, while the viscera, under pressure from the muscular walls of the abdomen, push the relaxed diaphragm back up into position. This reduces the thoracic and lung volume and increases the internal pressure, expelling from the lungs air that now contains less oxygen and more carbon dioxide and water vapor than when it entered them. The lungs, as a result of their elasticity, return to their original shape.

Our rhythmic breathing movements are usually made without any conscious interference at a rate of about 18 times per minute when at rest. Breathing in takes about a second and breathing out a little less than three seconds. Breathing is controlled by a region of the brain that is very sensitive to the concentration of carbon dioxide in the blood. If there is a rise in concentration, nerve impulses are sent automatically to the diaphragm and intercostal muscles to increase the rate and depth of breathing.

The *maximum*, or *vital*, *capacity* of the lungs is about 5 liters, but during quiet breathing the *tidal volume*, the volume of air moving in and out of the lungs, is between 500 and 750 ml. Furthermore, when we're breathing at rest, often the only active muscle is the diaphragm. Exercise increases the lung capacity. The vital capacity of a trained male athlete can be 6 liters or more. The greater the capacity of the lungs to expand and take in air, the greater the supply of oxygen for the vital functions of the body cells. During heavy exercise the tidal volume can be as much as 4.5 liters. This increase in oxygen intake helps increase the release of available energy for physical activity.

Energy and Energy Systems

The term *energy* refers to the capacity to do work or carry out physical activities. Energy is needed to maintain the body's temperature, to keep the heart beating and the lungs functioning, and to sustain all other bodily functions even when at rest. It is measured in either *calories* or *joules* (after the nineteenth-century British physicist J. P. Joule). Most popular books on diet and nutrition use the term *calories*, which in popular usage actually refers to kilocalories (the equivalent of 1,000 calories), because a calorie is a comparatively small measure.

(For a more complete explanation of joules and calories, see Appendix 2.) The amount of energy required to maintain the body at rest is referred to as the *basal metabolic rate* (BMR). Any movement or physical activity (including the additional energy required for growth, pregnancy, and lactation) beyond these basic body processes raises energy expenditure above the basal metabolic rate.

Energy is derived from the nutrients in our food, which are broken down and stored as chemical energy in body cells in the form of *adenosine triphosphate* (ATP). When a muscle contracts, ATP is broken down into *adenosine diphosphate* (ADP) and *phosphate*, releasing energy in the process. The amount of ATP stored in muscles is limited, so if energy is to continue to be released, ATP synthesis must keep pace with its consumption. To achieve this, the ADP molecule and its split-off phosphate are restored to ATP. This resynthesis requires energy, which is supplied through one of two energy systems: the *aerobic system* or the *anaerobic system*.

The Aerobic Energy System

Aerobic means working with air or, to be precise, oxygen. *Aerobics* refers to activities or exercises that allow muscles to work at a steady rate over an extended period of time with a continuous and adequate supply of oxygenated blood. The heart rate is increased by the activity to encourage the necessary blood supply. Aerobic activities can be sustained as long as the demand for oxygen to resynthesize ATP is satisfied.

Equally important are the sources of energy for the process. Carbohydrates are the main source of energy in our food. They are stored in the cells of the body in two usable forms, *glucose* and *glycogen*. (Glycogen is made of thousands of glucose molecules linked together.) *Cortisol*, a hormone produced by the adrenal glands, promotes the synthesis and storage of glucose. Glucose, sometimes referred to as *blood sugar*, is important to the normal functioning of the body; in fact, it is the only fuel used by the brain.

Aerobic activities use primarily glycogen and fatty acids as their sources of energy. Glycogen is stored in the muscle and liver. If the glycogen store is full, the excess is converted and stored as fat. Fat in the form of free fatty acids is stored in the *adipose* (fat) *tissue* and in skeletal muscle. These fatty acids can be mobilized for energy only by the aerobic energy system.

Generally, the release of energy in the body, whether aerobic or anaerobic, starts with the breakdown of glycogen into glucose and *pyruvates*. This process, called *glycolysis*, generates two molecules of ATP for each glucose molecule (see illustration on page 42). In aerobic respiration, the pyruvates then enter a cycle of reactions, usually

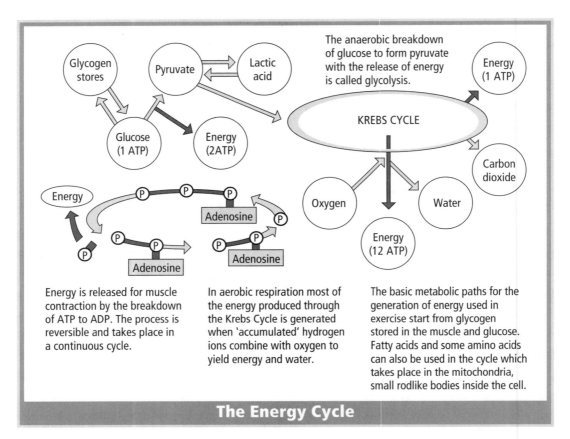

The anaerobic breakdown of glucose to form pyruvate with the release of energy is called glycolysis.

Energy is released for muscle contraction by the breakdown of ATP to ADP. The process is reversible and takes place in a continuous cycle.

In aerobic respiration most of the energy produced through the Krebs Cycle is generated when 'accumulated' hydrogen ions combine with oxygen to yield energy and water.

The basic metabolic paths for the generation of energy used in exercise start from glycogen stored in the muscle and glucose. Fatty acids and some amino acids can also be used in the cycle which takes place in the mitochondria, small rodlike bodies inside the cell.

The Energy Cycle

called the *Krebs cycle* after its discoverer, Sir Hans Krebs. The cycle of reactions is made possible by enzymes, with the assistance of coenzymes, which enable enzymes to do their work. Like all catalysts, the enzymes are not destroyed, but return to their original state after doing their specific chemical task, enabling the cycle to continue. Each "circuit" of the Krebs cycle yields one molecule of carbon dioxide and one molecule of ATP; it also "spins off" hydrogen ions that combine with oxygen to produce water and energy. It is this oxidation of the hydrogen

that releases most of the energy, 12 ATP molecules per cycle.

The entire process takes place in the cells within rod-shaped structures called *mitochondria*, where the enzymes that drive the Krebs cycle are found. For this reason the mitochondria are often called the cell's "powerhouse." Glucose is obtained from the blood and is drawn from the stores of glycogen. Fatty acids are also a source of energy; they are broken down into components that join directly into the Krebs cycle in the mitochondria. Although used continuously, fatty acids do not become a major source of energy until the body's carbohydrate resources are depleted. In extreme cases of starvation, when the body has insufficient carbohydrate or fat available, protein is also broken down to provide energy.

In practical terms, the use of glycogen and fat stores makes aerobic activities a vital tool for the control of body weight. If the objective is to reduce weight, an exercise program should be structured in its early stages around gentle, rhythmic exercises rather than high-intensity exercises that can take you outside the aerobic energy system to anaerobic energy systems (see below). The burning of fat generally takes place some 20 minutes from the start of the activity. Aerobic sessions of 20 to 30 minutes performed with moderate intensity at least three times a week can have tremendous health benefits. They improve stamina and endurance and strengthen the cardiovascular system. As mentioned previously, with improved conditioning the heart rate slows down both at rest and in activity, reducing stress to the organ. The stroke volume, the volume of blood pushed out per heartbeat, increases, reducing the work that the heart must do to circulate blood. The number of mitochondria also increases, improving the capacity of cells to use oxygen.

Anaerobic Energy Systems

Anaerobic energy systems produce energy without the use of oxygen. These systems come into use when the intensity of the activity is so great that the cardiorespiratory system cannot supply sufficient oxygen to meet the demands of the body. There are two different means of producing energy without oxygen: the lactate system and the creatine phosphate system.

The Lactate System

In physical exertion such as sprinting, the process of energy release stops at the first stage of the energy cycle, known as glycolysis, described earlier. Glycogen in the muscles is broken down to glucose to form *pyruvic acid* and to provide the energy required for the resynthesis of ATP. Glycolysis does not break down the glycogen completely and provides only a fraction of the ATP produced under the aerobic system. What is more, the end product of this anaerobic process is *lactic acid*, rather than water and carbon dioxide, the harmless products of the aerobic process. It is the accumulation of lactic acid in the muscles that causes fatigue, "stitch," cramps, and aches. The combined effect of this is that the intensity of the activity cannot be maintained for more than a matter of minutes. Fatigue may start to set in after 35 to 40 seconds and exhaustion after 55 to 60 seconds if the intensity of activity is high. Hence, the lactate system can only provide ATP energy for relatively short bursts of activity, such as for a 400-meter sprint, or for sprint finishes by middle- or long-distance runners. (These numbers are no more than approximate because the duration varies depending on the intensity of effort. If, for example, the sprint is done at 95 percent of the maximum intensity possible, the energy would be expended within 30 seconds.)

The Creatine Phosphate System

The body draws upon the creatine phosphate system when the energy requirement is so great that there is insufficient time to break down the glycogen to produce ATP energy. An example would be lifting very heavy weights. For this spurt of energy, the ADP stored in the muscle cells combines with creatine phosphate, which is also present, to provide energy for about 5 seconds of maximum effort. The reaction is reversible at rest when the level of ATP is relatively high. The recovery time depends on the intensity of effort and can range from 30 seconds after a 50 percent effort expenditure to 2 minutes following maximum effort. Although the energy from the creatine phosphate system is available for only a very short period, it can be drawn upon repeatedly because of the quick recovery of the supply.

A Comparison of Energy Systems

	Aerobic	Lactate	Creatine phosphate
Energy sources	Carbohydrates (glycogen), fats, and proteins	carbohydrates (glycogen and blood glucose)	creatine phosphate
Level of activity	low intensity	high intensity	extremely high
Examples of sport/activity	walking, long-distance running, swimming	sustained sprint, uphill running	short sprint, weight lifting, squash
Duration*	varies, but normally for hours if level of intensity is low	varies depending on intensity; maximum duration within minutes	seconds
Recovery time	varies depending on glycogen availability	varies, but less than 2 hours	full recovery in 2 minutes
Waste products	carbon dioxide and water	lactic acid	none

*approximation depending on the individual and the effort exerted

How Energy Systems Relate to Exercise

Most sports and exercises use a combination of energy systems (see table on the previous page). In an exercise-to-music class, for example, the warm-up would use movements involving the big muscle groups in a series of low-impact and traveling moves to raise the heartbeat and increase the supply of blood to muscles. This would involve the aerobic energy system, but after a period of increased heart activity of 10 to 15 minutes, the workout could increase in intensity to a level where the energy requirement begins to exceed that provided by the aerobic system, for example in a series of explosive movements such as high kicks and jumping jacks. The anaerobic energy system would then come into play. Certainly the lactate system would set in, at least intermittently, if the class were to move on to training activities for strengthening muscles, during which the heart rate would be brought down even further.

In general, exercises that concentrate on building strength tend to rely principally on anaerobic energy while those that focus on endurance rely on aerobic energy. Hence, it is technically incorrect to refer to exercise-to-music classes as *aerobics*. Circuit classes also tend to combine aerobic with anaerobic energy use. Soccer players use both aerobic and anaerobic energy systems. Even when jogging, different energy systems can be brought into play in different terrains. However, some exercise regimes use more of one energy system than the other. This may have a crucial influence on what types of exercise are chosen to meet specific objectives. (Chapter 5 reviews in more detail the different exercise regimes available.)

4

Setting Sensible Targets for Exercise

People take up sports or exercise for many reasons. The most common ones are to meet other people, to improve health and fitness, to prepare for a particular sport or activity, and for enjoyment and relaxation. The objectives for improving health and fitness vary significantly from person to person. Some hope to gain greater strength, others seek increased stamina, while yet others want to lose weight, reshape their body, or increase flexibility. Very often, people in sedentary occupations go to the gym for a hard workout in order to remove surplus energy and to find relief from the dullness and stress of their working day. A common goal, particularly among middle-aged men, is to increase cardiovascular and respiratory fitness. Increasingly, people use exercise as a way of gaining tranquillity and calmness, and as a cure for anxiety, restlessness, and sleeplessness. Most people, however, seek a combination of these objectives with greater or less emphasis on one or the other. Whatever the specific objectives, the final overall target is to feel healthier and to look better.

Understanding our body is essential if we are to set sensible objectives for ourselves. In Chapter 3, we learned that the makeup of our muscles bears an important influence on what we can do. From the information given on bone structure and bone formation, we learned the importance of weight-bearing activities and joint mobility. The coverage on energy systems illustrated the importance of aerobic training for cardiovascular health and weight control. However, other influences come into play, particularly what might be described as our natural endowments, in the search to understand what exercise and sports can or cannot achieve.

Body Shape or Somatotype

The basic shape of a person is determined by hereditary or genetic factors, nutrition, environment, and culture. Much controversy has surrounded the subject of how much of what we are is determined by the environment and how much by genetic factors: the age-old argument of nature versus nurture. Over the lifetime of a single generation, hereditary and genetic factors undoubtedly have an overwhelming influence on body type. Our genetic inheritance greatly determines how we look. In fact, human populations can be categorized or distinguished by some genetic differences, including blood type and even susceptibility to some kinds of disease.

Taken over many generations, environmental factors such as climate and food patterns have had an impact on the genetic constitution of humanity. Human evolution has demonstrated the influence of different environmental conditions. People tend to be tall and thin in very hot climates because a larger surface area relative to body mass allows for greater heat loss. Thus, African groups such as the Nilotes have probably the highest ratio of surface to body mass. In cold climates the reverse is true; people tend to be short and stocky, thereby reducing the surface-to-mass ratio. The Inuits of the Arctic region are prime examples. In climates with intense sunshine, the iris is deeply pigmented to reduce the impact of injurious ultraviolet light on the eye. Studies on how humans are adapted to their environment have shown a direct link between levels of sunlight and pigmentation.

Access to different foods under different climates also influences body form. Although body measurements are linked to hereditary/genetic factors, they are also affected by nutrition. Better-nourished people tend to grow larger because an improved diet allows for the building of greater bone and muscle mass. A feature of emigration is that the children of people who as a rule are short may grow surprisingly tall in their new homeland.

The physical differences that emerge as a result of geography, climate, and nutrition help to explain why within each of the broad racial groups—Caucasoid, Negroid, and Mongoloid—such wide differences in build and facial features can develop. Africans south of the Sahara are characterized by heavy concentrations of melanin in the skin,

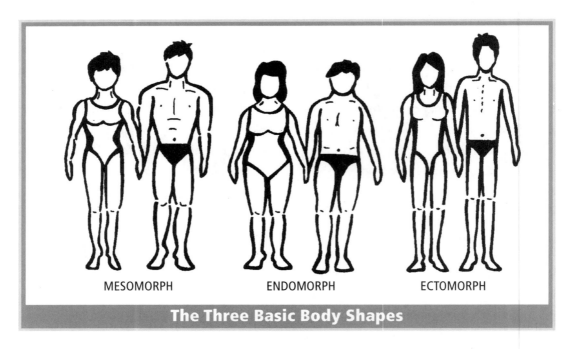

MESOMORPH   ENDOMORPH   ECTOMORPH

The Three Basic Body Shapes

while those in Ethiopia and Somalia, towards the Gulf of Aden, and in the Cape area in the far south have less pigmentation. In fact, such diversity has made the rigid demarcation of racial groups into Caucasoid, Negroid, and Mongoloid untenable. This is reinforced by DNA analysis, which reveals very little genetic difference among the peoples of the world.

Setting aside any consideration of human evolution or racial groups, the human body can be broadly categorized into three types: *ectomorph*, *endomorph*, and *mesomorph* (see illustration above). People classified as ectomorphs usually have a long, lean frame and narrow shoulders and hips. Long-distance runners often fall into this category. Endomorphs, by contrast, are short and broad, with wide hips and a tendency to gain weight. Mesomorphs are athletic in build with broad shoulders, narrow waist, and powerful, but not wide, hips. Gymnasts and sprinters are often this shape.

The basic shape or skeletal framework of a person, whether ectomorph, mesomorph, endomorph, or a combination (few people fall neatly into one specific category), cannot be changed by exercise. Exercise and food intake, however, can influence how you look. A mesomorph who takes no exercise and overeats can look like an endomorph. An endomorph can, through sensible exercise and eating habits, acquire a toned body that is significantly more fit than that of a mesomorph who leads a sedentary life. Even if you are born with what current fashion dictates as the "right" body type, this does not necessarily mean it will be easy to maintain. It is vital to start the pursuit of health and fitness at an early age through good nutritional habits and regular exercise. Although everyone is born with a basic shape, a great deal can be done to influence how it looks and, equally important, how one feels about one's physical appearance, health, and fitness.

Keeping the Body Ticking

As mentioned in Chapter 3, the energy needed to keep the body functioning at rest and in a fasting state is called the *basal metabolic rate* (BMR). This includes the energy required for breathing, heartbeat, maintenance of nerve functions, secretions from body glands and cells, body temperature, and tension in muscles. In short, it is the minimum energy required to sustain life.

The BMR varies from person to person depending on body weight, height, body composition, age, environmental factors, and sex. Muscles are metabolically more active than fat; therefore, a muscular person will have a higher BMR than a person with the same weight but a higher fat content. Women, whose bodies naturally have a higher fat content than men, have a lower BMR. A tall thin person with a large body surface relative to her/his weight will have a higher BMR than a short thin person because of the greater loss of heat and the need to maintain body temperature. If, however, the ambient temperature is greater than the body temperature (36.5°C, or 98.6°F), the reverse is true, because the larger surface area of the tall thin person's body allows greater absorption of heat, reducing the need for energy to maintain body temperature. In hot climates the BMR of any individual, whether fat or thin, is generally 10 to 20 percent lower than it would be if they were living in a temperate climate.

The BMR on a per-unit-weight basis generally declines with age, as the composition of the body changes. It is highest on a per-unit-weight basis in young children during the growth spurts associated with puberty (between 10 and 15 years of age), when more energy is required for bone formation and growth. At a later stage in adulthood, the BMR generally declines at about 2 percent per year. If a person were to maintain the same food intake and physical activity in old age as when young, there would be an inevitable gain in weight. During sleep the BMR is lowered. Interestingly, the BMR is lowered when people on a slimming diet reduce their food intake, because muscle as well as fat tissue is lost. Women who are lactating or pregnant have a higher BMR.

The BMR in calories can be calculated, using a simplified formula, by multiplying body weight in kilograms by 0.9 (for women) or 1.0 (for men) and then by 24 (the hours in a day). Thus, a woman who weighs 63 kg will have an estimated BMR of 63 x 0.9 x 24 = 1,361 calories (to determine your weight in kilograms, divide your weight in pounds by 2.2046; thus, a body weight of 140 pounds equals 63.5 kg). This is only an approximation, because height, muscle tone, and age also affect the BMR. Using different formulae in the calculation also produces different approximations. Appendix 1 provides examples of the different methods that can be used to estimate the BMR. See also the table titled "Average BMR...," on page 54, for a general guideline on BMR, taking into account sex, age, and height.

While the BMR is the minimum energy needed to sustain life, energy is also required for the digestion of food, absorption of nutrients, and for coping with sudden changes in temperature, emotion, and stress—cumulatively referred to as *facultative thermogenesis*. Additional energy is also needed for physical activities. The sum total of all these (BMR, facultative thermogenesis, and physical activities) makes up our total energy need.

Metabolism is the sum of all the chemical reactions within the body, whether involving the breakdown of substances such as glycogen, or the synthesis of complex substances such as proteins. The *metabolic rate* is a measure of the energy used in these processes. Metabolism includes both the catabolic and anabolic processes. A *catabolic* process is one in which a complex substance is broken into simpler ones for the release of energy, for example, when glucose is broken down into water and carbon dioxide. An *anabolic* process is one in which a complex substance is built up from simpler substances, such as the synthesis of complex proteins from amino acids.

The metabolic rate increases following food consumption, following exertion, during fluctuations in temperature, and during emotional stress or illness. Digestion alone can use as much as 5–10 percent of the calorie intake. The metabolic rate is controlled principally by hormones (such as adrenaline, noradrenaline, insulin, thyroid hormones, and corticosteroid hormones), which influence the chemical processes within the body.

During exercise, the metabolic rate is raised. Sustained exercise also increases the BMR, which can stay some 10 percent above its normal level for up to 48 hours after the exercise has ceased. This postexercise elevation of BMR contributes to fat loss, especially when exercise is performed on a regular and sustained basis. Exercise also raises the BMR over time by increasing the body's muscle.

Food and Diet

The metabolic rate is only one side of the equation determining body weight. Whether the body increases in weight depends on the caloric value of food consumed relative to energy expenditure—or in other words, how much you eat compared to how much you move. Food intake in excess of what the body needs leads to weight gain through the storage of fat, and eventually to obesity.

Fat is stored in *adipose tissue* (located in a layer just beneath the skin); around internal organs, including the heart, kidneys, and liver; and in the abdominal walls. Left to accumulate, this fat is not only unattractive but poses several health risks, increasing the risk of hypertension, heart disease, stroke, diabetes, and gallstones. In men, adipose tissue tends to accumulate around the shoulders, waist, and abdomen; in women, it tends to lodge in the breasts, hips, and thighs. Dr. Pamela Peeke, of the U.S. National Institutes of Health, found in a study on the link between stress and fat that both men and women, when under persistent mental stress, tend to accumulate fat in the abdominal walls.[4] Stress raises the levels of cortisol in the blood, resulting in a surge in appetite and a search for comfort foods. (Cortisol is a hormone produced by the adrenal glands.)

Many factors influence the accumulation of fat in the body. Some people tend to gain weight more easily than others at a given level of food intake. This might be attributed to a lower BMR. Hereditary factors can play a part. It is also possible that in some cases the weight problem is created because parents pass on bad eating habits to their children.

Persistent overconsumption of food, especially food rich in fat and sugar, can cause *hypertrophy*, wherein the existing fat cells increase in size, or *hyperplasia*, wherein the number of fat cells increase. Once the number of fat cells has risen, it cannot be reduced. By contrast, the size of fat cells is reducible. The foundation for the development of number of fat cells is believed to be laid down in three phases: before birth, between one and two years, and in adolescence. The subject is still controversial, however, because the propensity to gain weight varies so widely between people. Despite a lack of consensus, there is general agreement on the importance of balancing calorie consumption with energy expenditure, although the "balance" seems to differ from person to person.

The table on page 52 contains a table of selected foods and their caloric equivalent in physical activity. The table is not a guide on how to "spend" the calories contained in the foods you consume, but rather demonstrates how difficult it is to achieve a balance in energy expenditure and consumption in the face of persistent overeating. It is estimated that to lose a single pound of fat, 3,500 calories must be expended. The table titled "Average Energy Expended...," on page 53, provides a summary of the average energy expenditure of everyday activities at home, in the workplace, and at leisure.

Between the ages of 25 and 50 years, an average *recommended daily allowance* (RDA) of 2,200 calories is required by women and 2,900 calories by men to sustain life and carry out normal activity. This estimate is derived by multiplying the BMR by a factor of 1.6, assuming moderate physical activity, and then adjusted upwards for younger people and downwards for older people. For those engaged in high levels of physical activity, the daily calorie in-

take is substantially more. If the level of physical activity is higher than "average," then a factor of 1.8 is applicable. Athletes engaged in regular training for cross-country skiing, cycling, or marathon running may need even more calories (see the table on page 189). In the United Kingdom, on the other hand, the factor used in the calculation of the average requirements for energy is 1.4, because of an underlying assumption that on average people have a comparatively sedentary lifestyle with little physical activity at work and at leisure. The United Kingdom's *estimated average requirement* (EAR) of energy has also been incorporated into the table titled "Average BMR...,"on page 54, to illustrate the influence on energy requirements of a sedentary

Caloric Content of Selected Foods and Duration of Activities Required for Their Utilization*

Food	Calories	Walking 2 mph	Jogging 5.5 mph	Aerobic dancing	Swimming (slow crawl) 2 mph
Apple (4.5 oz.), medium	40	16 minutes	5 minutes	7 minutes	10 minutes
Rump steak (3.5 oz.), fried	224	93 minutes	26 minutes	38 minutes	57 minutes
Roast chicken with skin (3.5 oz.)	244	102 minutes	28 minutes	42 minutes	62 minutes
Bread (one slice)	60	25 minutes	7 minutes	10 minutes	15 minutes
Baked potato	170	71 minutes	20 minutes	29 minutes	43 minutes

* The figures are all approximate based on a person weighing 110 pounds and working at low intensity and effort. The greater the body weight, the more calories consumed; the greater the effort, the more calories consumed.

Average Energy Expended in Everyday Activities and Selected Sports

Calories/minute		Calories/minute		Calories/minute	
Everyday activities		**Sports**		**Sports** (cont'd.)	
sitting	1.4	aerobics, heavy	8	jogging (1 mile/15 min.)	5
standing	1.7	aerobics, moderate	5	rowing (11 mph)	13
washing/dressing	3.5	aerobics, light	3	running (1 mile/5 min.)	18
walking slowly	3	badminton, doubles	4	running (1 mile/7 min.)	13.5
walking moderately quickly	5	badminton, singles	5.1	swimming, fast	9.4
walking up and down stairs/hills	9	bowling	3.9	swimming, slow	7.7
		calisthenics, light	4	tennis, doubles	5.0
At work		cycling (6 mph)	3.5	tennis, singles	6.5
light (most domestic work)	.5–4.9	cycling (10 mph)	5.5	volleyball	5.1
moderate (gardening)	5.0	cycling (12 mph)	7.5		
strenuous (coal mining)	7.5	jogging (1 mile/9 min.)	10		

* The figures are all approximate based on a person weighing 110 pounds and working at low intensity and effort. The greater the body weight, the more calories consumed; the greater the effort, the more calories consumed.

(Source: Ministry of Agriculture, Fisheries, and Food. *Manual of Nutrition*. Her Majesty's Stationery Office, 1992; data on sports activities from First DataBank data, Hearst Corporation, 1994.)

lifestyle. It should be noted, however, that part of the difference between the EAR established in the United Kingdom and the RDA set in the United States and elsewhere is the product of differences in weight and height in the population samples used. The RDA figures are the ones used by the Food and Agriculture Organization (FAO) and the World Health Organization's (WHO) Consultative Group on Nutrition. It should be stressed that important differences in RDA exist depending upon climate, temperature, geography, and people.

In general, restricting food intake to a level greatly below what the body requires is a dubious way of losing weight. Starving sends confusing signals to the body, and as a result the body's cells will respond by storing energy once the dieter returns to regular eating habits. In addition, weight lost during this kind of extreme dieting consists of both fat and lean body mass, resulting in a lowering of the BMR. As a result, less energy is spent on maintaining body functions and more is left over for storage. Reducing food intake can also cause depression and anxiety.

	Age	Weight (lbs.)	Height (inches)	BMR cal/day	RDA cal/day	EAR cal/day
Average BMR, RDA of Energy in the U.S., and EAR of Energy in the U.K., by Gender/Age for Sample Gender/Age/Weight/Height Categories						
Male	11–14	99	62	1,440	2,500	2,220
	15–18	145	69	1,760	3,000	2,755
	19–24	154	70	1,780	2,900	2,550
	25–50	175	69	1,800	2,900	2,550
	51+	170	68	1,530	2,300	2,340
Female	11–14	100	62	1,310	2,200	1,845
	15–18	120	64	1,370	2,200	2,110
	19–24	128	64.5	1,350	2,200	1,940
	25–50	139	64	1,380	2,200	1,940
	51+	143	63	1,280	1,900	1,880

(Source: *Recommended Dietary Allowance.* Washington, DC: National Academy Press, 1989; Dietary Reference Values for Food Energy and Nutrients for the United Kingdom, London: Her Majesty's Stationery Office, 1991.)

A combination of sensible food intake and regular exercise offers a much more viable route to weight loss. Exercise stimulates the release in the brain of *endorphins*, natural painkillers with a chemical structure similar to morphine that induce a sense of well-being. They also help to counteract the influence of the hormone cortisol, moderating the desire for food. In fact, studies have shown that a modest increase in the intensity of exercise may be mirrored by a decrease in appetite and food consumption (see Chapter 12 for more on food and nutrition).

Spot Reduction of Fat

Body fat is not evenly distributed. There are particular areas where it tends to accumulate. For women, bottoms and tummies are not the only areas of concern. Flabby underarms and the buildup of fat in the inner and outer thighs are just as worrying. For men, the so-called "love handles" and "beer bellies" very often go hand in hand with age. People can be classified into apple and pear shapes according to where the fat accumulates. The apple shape is associated with upper-body obesity and the pear shape with lower-body obesity. However, this division can have implications beyond mere shape. Apple-shaped people seem to be more susceptible to hypertension, coronary diseases, and diabetes than pear-shaped ones. One explanation may be that the higher metabolic activity that accompanies abdominal fat results in higher levels of fat in the blood. Another is the sedentary lifestyle often associated with pot-bellies.

The tendency of fat to accumulate in specific parts of the body means that, for many people, the objective of a workout is to concentrate on reducing the fat in one part of their body. This, however, is a highly controversial topic. Many specialists are of the view that such spot reduction is not feasible because the loss of fat is not point specific.

While the general thrust of this argument is logical, it is not altogether accurate to say that exercise has no spot-reduction effect. Aerobic exercises draw fat from wherever it is located. While this may mean that the fat is not drawn initially from the target areas, with time, patience, and perseverance this specific fat can eventually be used by the body. An argument can also be made that with regular exercise muscles become stronger and better toned. A bottom that is toned looks different from one that is flabby, even if its size remains unchanged. Here, strength-building (toning) exercises

play a significant part. It is important to stress that strength-building regimes need to be complemented by aerobic activities if they are to be effective. More about these topics are covered in Chapters 7 and 8.

Getting Older

Aging is inevitable. How we age is determined by hereditary factors and lifestyle. In general, a progressive physiological decline occurs. The efficiency of the body's organs—including the heart, kidneys, lungs, and liver—declines. The skin loses elasticity, causing it to sag, wrinkle, and bruise easily. Muscles lose bulk and strength. Reflexes slow as muscle fibers change, with a reduction in fast-twitch fibers. Postural muscles shorten. Bones become more porous and joints become less stable as a result of wear and tear. The pressure exerted on the intervertebral discs compresses them, resulting in a loss of height. The senses of smell, touch, and hearing become less sharp as nerve cells decline in number. The loss of brain cells reduces the ability to acquire new skills. Resistance to disease and the capacity for body repair decline. These degenerative processes are accelerated by an excessive consumption of alcohol, drugs, and food, by poor diet, smoking tobacco, environmental pollution, a lack of exercise, sports injuries, and so on. There is also a tendency for the BMR to fall and body weight to rise.

Exercise can help slow down some of the degenerative processes. With regular exercise, an old person can retain a large proportion of his/her strength and stamina. Muscles are seldom lost unless through disease and lack of use. The ability to maintain strength and endurance helps preserve physical performance. The intensity of the exercises, however, might have to be reduced because of decreased lung capacity.

The extent and speed of decline varies from person to person, and the sports arena abounds with examples of fit 60-year-olds. In the book *Survival of the Fittest*, Mike Stroud describes the phenomenal prowess of Helen Klein, one of the greatest long-distance runners in the world. When they met she was 72 years old and had recently joined a team competing in Eco-Challenge, a long-distance race that involved crossing more than 300 miles of the southwestern United States, using a combination of running, horseback riding, mountain biking, and hiking.[5] She first took up long-distance running at age 55; by the time she joined the team for Eco-Challenge at 72, she had completed 75 marathons and 150 ultramarathons and was still capable of running 100 miles in twenty hours. While not everyone can be a Helen Klein, and jogging might well be suitable for some and not others, regular exercise, especially begun early in life, contributes to the maintenance of cardiorespiratory fitness, muscular strength, and endurance when older.

Gender Differences

People vary because of differences in their anatomy and physiology. Differences may relate to factors such as race, geographical location, climate, food, age, and livelihood. But nowhere are differences more obvious and significant than those related to gender. The differences between men and women have to be understood before appropriate training or exercise regimes and targets can be set.

In terms of anatomy, if we were to consider an average man and woman, the man would have broader shoulders, longer arms, and greater upper-body strength. He would also have longer legs, narrower hips, and a smaller slant of the femur. He would be taller. His body would contain 42 percent muscle and between 12 and 14 percent fat, compared with the woman's 36 percent muscle and 20–24 percent fat. The man's body would contain 4 percent more water than the woman's.

Anatomical differences already make the man a more efficient runner, with a longer stride and more powerful muscular output. The wider pelvis of the woman makes it difficult to bring the knees close together, making running more difficult.

The Achilles tendon in the woman is also shorter and tighter, impairing takeoff. But the man also has other important advantages, with a larger heart, larger stroke volume and cardiac output, greater blood volume (some 5–6 liters compared to 4–4.5 liters in the woman), larger volume of body fluid, larger lungs (by some 10 percent), and a higher respiratory and ventilation rate. The hemoglobin count in a woman is 10 percent lower than in a man with the same volume of blood. Oxygen uptake is more efficient in the man and some 15–20 percent higher than in the woman, allowing the man a greater release of energy to power the muscles. The woman, however, has greater joint mobility and greater flexibility in her muscles.

The reproductive physiology of women must also be taken into consideration. Strenuous training can disrupt the menstrual cycle in a number of ways. The onset of menstruation, which usually occurs around the age of 12, is often delayed in girls training for events such as gymnastics, dance, and swimming. For those already menstruating, ovulation and menstruation can be disrupted. *Amenorrhea* (the absence of menstrual periods, sometimes with gaps of 6 months to a year) is not considered dangerous in itself, but may have an adverse effect on the bone structure. The lowering of estrogen levels in the blood that arises as a result of amenorrhea reduces the deposition of calcium phosphate in the bones. Osteoporosis weakens the bones and increases the risk of bone injury. In young athletes a failure to lay down sufficient calcium phosphates in the early years of development increases the problem of osteoporosis in menopause. Intense training can also contribute to increased injuries because the hormonal changes during the menstrual cycle affect bones, muscles, and tendons that are already being subjected to intense stress.

The anatomical and physiological differences between men and women clearly affect athletic performance. Men, with their greater aerobic capacity, strength, and endurance, have a clear advantage in power sports and activities such as running. Women have an advantage in physical regimes that require mobility and flexibility, such as floor gymnastics. These are important factors determining the formulation of exercise regimes and should be applied even to body-conditioning exercises. This subject is covered in some more detail in Chapter 8, which deals with training for muscular strength and endurance.

5

Fusion Fitness: The Broad Approach to Exercise

Like fashion, exercise regimes for improving fitness, health, and beauty have gone through tremendous changes over the years. In the 1970s and '80s, the hard workout with its famous "burn" was all the rage. It gave rise to high-energy, high-impact moves in aerobic training. People preferred these classes because they were associated with a certain level of fitness and, in a sense, status. Muscular- and endurance-training programs similarly focused on big movements that allowed people to take joints and muscles to their "full range" of movement. Once again, they were executed in an energetic way, with arms and legs swinging in great arcs. Sit-ups were done rapidly. Squats were deep, taking the buttocks well below knee level. Weights were incorporated into workouts. Explosive movements were in vogue, and stretches were often ballistic. The saying "no pain, no gain" became the password of the cognoscenti.

Widespread incidences of injuries as well as improvements in sports science over the past decade or so have modified the view that pace and burn are everything. Gradually, high-impact aerobics, although still popular, is giving way to combinations of high and low movements, encouraged perhaps by the growing number of people in their middle and later years now taking up exercise.

In the building of muscle strength and endurance, two contrasting "new" trends are being superimposed on the old ones. The first is a modified traditional approach that continues to focus on promoting the full range of movements in joints and muscles, but remains cautious. All positions that require extreme flexion have been taken off the list of recommended exercises. For example, while touching the toes from an upright position was once an almost universal exercise in school PE classes, it is now considered dangerous. The fear that class participants may hurt themselves has led instructors to avoid any possibility of danger. "Do not work through pain" has now become the motto.

The second development, running parallel to this cautious approach, incorporates little or no aerobic training. It includes exercise disciplines initiated by Lotte Berk, as well as those generally classified as *callanetics*. In these systems, exercise techniques are especially focused on getting into the right position before beginning any movement, and movements are slow and controlled.

Lotte Berk's method, based on her experience with dance and later with orthopedic exercises, promoted awareness of joints and especially the spine. Her knowledge of orthopedic methods was acquired during her recovery from a spinal injury caused by an accident. Some of the positions she taught did require extreme flexion of the body, but getting into them involved first getting the joints stable and controlled. The "rolling in of the pelvis," for example, was a cornerstone of her abdominal exercises. Movements varied from full range to smaller ones, but all were difficult: Just getting into the right position could take weeks of practice. The barre, traditionally limited to use by ballet dancers, was a prerequisite tool for supporting some of the positions.

Developed and refined by Callan Pinckney, who had trained under Lotte Berk, callanetics is in many ways similar to Berk's style of exercise. The two methods differ from one another in two primary ways. In callanetics, almost all the movements are small; additionally, some of the movements are very repetitive, with targets for abdominal contractions, for example, set at 100 reps. Muscle groups are isolated, and their small, almost imperceptible movements are consistently applied as though against an invisible and immovable resistance.

While these two disciplines gained widespread support in some quarters, they were less accepted in others. Amongst those training for sports and athletics, there emerged a trend away from *isometric training*, i.e., the practice of developing muscle tension without changing muscle length. When that happened, exercises involving small movements that facilitated such muscle tension became less popular because of their similarities to isometric training.

Isometric training for weight lifting, which had been all the rage previously, also declined.[6] While isometric contractions are useful as a rehabilitative exercise for developing strength in specific places on the body, they must be used with caution because of potential adverse results, of which raised blood pressure ranks as one of the most serious. (Chapter 8 discusses in greater detail the advantages and disadvantages of isometric training.) In athletic training today, as opposed to in the general fitness industry, isometric exercises are rarely practiced except in conjunction with other training methods.

More recently, holistic exercise regimes have been added to the fitness brew. Stress and strife in the modern industrialized world have encouraged a search for nature and tranquillity. Just as homeopathic medicines have revived in popularity and organic foods are a must for many consumers, yoga, t'ai chi, Pilates, the Alexander Technique, and a host of other similar forms of holistic exercise have become either popular or have revived in popularity in the West. Their practitioners consider them holistic or complete because they involve both the mind and the body. Some, such as t'ai chi and yoga, have their origins in antiquity. By returning to age-old traditions, practices such as t'ai chi and yoga offer a sense of security during times of rapid societal change. Some people question, however, whether such regimes have lost some of their original intent in the transition from one very different culture to another.

Holistic Regimes

Yoga

Yoga has been practiced for literally thousands of years in India. The word itself means "union with God." As in the eight-fold path of Buddhism, there are eight components to the achievement of this union as prescribed by Patanjali, the father of yoga. The first concerns moral disciplines; the second personal disciplines of purity, devotion to God, study, and contentment; the third and fourth revolve around the practice of posture and breath control; the fifth through eighth involve the practice of concentration—meditation to allow the mind to become quiet, thereby allowing the person to discover pure consciousness, a oneness with the universe. These components form the wheel of yoga, which makes up all aspects of living—a complete way of life.

Two main schools predominate in the modern practice of yoga:

- *Hatha yoga* focuses on the more physical aspects, such as postures based principally on the stretching movements of animals, and breath control.

- *Raja yoga* teaches concentration, meditation, and discovery of oneness with the universe, a sense of withdrawal.

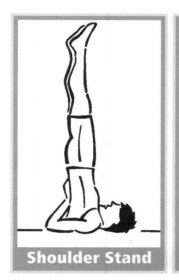

Shoulder Stand

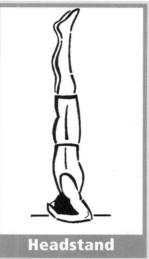

Headstand

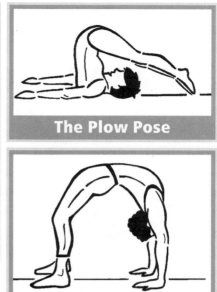

The Plow Pose

Back Arch Pose

In the Western world, hatha yoga has the most appeal. For many, yoga is a means to relax, to overcome stress, to increase flexibility, and to have greater body control. In effect, it has become an exercise regime.

As an exercise regime, especially in flexibility training, yoga has much to offer. Its use of breath control to get into the various postures (*asanas*) helps to relax the body, and relaxed muscles are easier to stretch than tight ones. Greater awareness of the body is promoted through concentration. The stretches or postures are done symmetrically, which illustrates an understanding of balanced muscle development. A forward bend is complemented by a backward bend; a stretch to the left is followed by one to the right. Given that yoga originated long before sports science was born, this is remarkable. Practices such as

the use of "recti breathing" techniques to isolate the abdominal muscle and retraction abdominal controls were only recently recognized in the sports world, giving rise to the so-called abdominal revolution, the concept of *core stability*, and Pilates.

Not all yoga positions are suitable for all people. In fact, some positions, I believe, can be dangerous.[7] Remember from Chapter 3 that muscles work in pairs; for each movement, there's a set of muscles acting as agonist and another as antagonist. In many yoga postures the muscles involved are contracted and stretched, i.e., one set of muscles is contracting to "hold" the stretch of the opposing muscle group. Yoga stretches are generally held for a significant length of time—much longer than the 25- to 30- second hold typical of developmental stretches, and certainly much longer than the holds generally recommended for active stretches, which is the category of stretching to which many of the yoga postures belong (see Chapter 10 for a description of active stretches). It is suggested in yoga, for example, that headstands and shoulder stands are held for some minutes, with the knees kept very straight and the spine and legs kept elongated upward.[8] Holding such an unchanged posture would involve the tensing of the agonist muscle, without much change in the length of the muscle fibers. In inverted postures such as headstands (*Sirisana*), shoulder stands (*Sarvangasana*), the plow pose (*Halasana*), and the wheel or back arch pose (*Chakrasana*) (see figures on page 61), blood rushes not only to the head but also to the heart, which needs to contract with much greater force to drive blood through the circulatory system, increasing both its systolic and diastolic pressure.

Many people pursue such postures in the belief that they are beneficial for health. The plow pose is supposed to tone the nervous system, stimulate the endocrine glands, liver, and spleen, correct menstrual disorder, prevent disorders of the stomach, and "normalize" obesity. Shoulder stands supposedly increase the sexual fitness of both men and women, reduce excess fat,

and soothe and tone the nervous system.[9] These claims need scientific verification at the least, and in the case of individuals with hypertension, these postures could actually be risky. Inverted postures carry with them yet another possible risk, namely the considerable pressure and weight exerted on the spine. This danger is magnified in the case of overweight individuals.

In the plow pose and shoulder stands the pressure is on the cervical spine, just at the back of the neck and base of the head. This is an important center for the nervous network. Even when the body is supported with the hands, the cervical vertebrae are engaged in an acute angle and subjected to compression by the weight they have to bear from the body when it is centered directly above. In shoulder stands, gravity would most likely offset any stretch or "lengthening" of the spine. To hold the position, muscles must contract rather than relax. In the back arch the small of the back is compressed, and the neck muscle is either isometrically contracted to keep the chin toward the chest (the recommended position) or hyperextended when it hangs back; the wrists are also subject to the substantial weight of the body. In headstands the shoulders and elbows carry most of the body weight, for which they are not suited. Some noninverted postures, such as the peacock (see figure on the next page), are similarly stressful for the wrists.

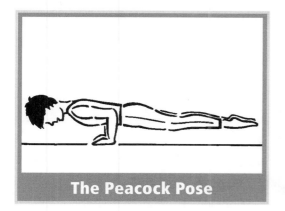

The Peacock Pose

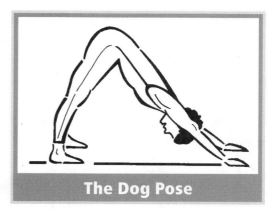

The Dog Pose

In some of the forward poses, the problem of extreme flexion is met to an extent by yogic breathing techniques and abdominal-muscle control. They allow practitioners to bend without experiencing the pressure that otherwise would be exerted on the joints. A good example is the dog pose (see figure above), where, by holding in the stomach, much of the pressure on the back is removed. It is for this reason that some of the forward-bending yoga postures have been adopted and modified to feature in the stretching positions of the sports and fitness world. With the correct techniques of breathing and abdominal-muscle control, and with the modification of the postures to exclude movements that take joints beyond their natural range, more of these stretches could be used.

Thus, as an exercise regime, yoga offers benefits that include flexibility training and muscle control, but it is not a complete program of fitness. It provides little aerobic training, which is important for cardiovascu-

lar benefits as well as weight control, and involves virtually no or very limited motor-skill development in terms of eye–limb response and coordination. Its relaxation and withdrawal techniques are useful for coping with stress, but it is not a technique that can be easily applied, for example, in the workplace where the stress occurs. Most importantly, some of the postures could be dangerous.

T'ai Chi Chuan

T'ai chi chuan is a Chinese martial art that dates back to the early third century A.D. By the fifth century, t'ai chi chuan had become a key form of martial art and exercise in the Buddhist monastery of Shao Lin.

The term *t'ai chi* has been variously translated as "great gargantuan fist," "great polarity boxing," and "shadowboxing." There is in fact no single definition, because it is an art form that has been modified and changed with time. The only central intrinsic concept is the idea of internal energy or "chi" (sometimes spelled *qi*). Chi is derived from three sources: There is the chi we are born with, the chi we obtain from food, and the chi derived from breathing. The last is central to the physical regime because the reservoir of chi is believed to lie in the stomach. The thrust is, therefore, to breathe using the "stomach," or diaphragm, to replenish our energy levels.

This belief cuts across practically all Chinese martial arts and methods for healing. In fact, the practice of breath control in China dates to the period from 221 B.C. to A.D. 906, when Taoism flourished. The Taoists developed breathing techniques called *qi gong* (pronounced and sometimes spelled, "chi kung") to control the flow of energy in the body. Used also to preserve and regulate the flow of semen, for healing, and in martial arts, qi gong has revived in popularity in recent years. In Chinese acupressure, the point lying three fingers' width below the navel is referred to as the "sea of energy." In t'ai chi this is known as *tan tien*.

In t'ai chi the body is considered a unified entity and the tan tien is the center of movement, with the arms and legs mere extensions of it. Belief in these vital points of energy is shared by practitioners of other Far Eastern disciplines, such as Japanese shiatsu and Thai massage.

As a means of attack or defense, t'ai chi is practiced both with and without weapons. As an exercise discipline it seeks to promote health and relaxation through body conditioning that involves smooth, deliberate, and rhythmic movements with carefully choreographed positions and stances. The stances emulate the movements of the bear, deer, monkey, tiger, snake, and bird. Most of the movements are performed slowly, interspersed with occasional fast and rapid moves that might imitate, for example, an animal in flight.

Balance, coordination, and breathing control are required. The entire body is involved in the movements, including the eye, face (for example, in raising the eyebrow), arms, legs, torso, hands, fingers, feet, and toes. All movements flow from one to another without any break, and depending on the school or the master there can be from 24 to over 100 prescribed exercise forms or chapters. Total concentration and quiet is required. The ability to complete the prescribed chapters requires considerable memory power and patience. The underlying principle that binds the movements is the harmonization of the two important forces of the universe, the *yin* (passive, female) and the *yang* (active, male). When they are in balance, equilibrium, peace, and harmony are believed to have been achieved.

Many schools of t'ai chi chuan have existed; of these, two remain today, the Wu and the Yang. In China, the discipline is handed down from master to student, and no master teaches the system exactly like another because the choreography has a

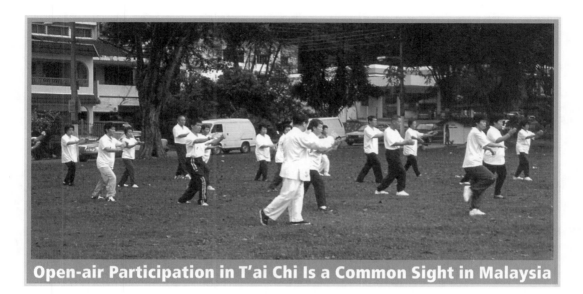

Open-air Participation in T'ai Chi Is a Common Sight in Malaysia

story as its underlying base. There are, however, common moves based on the movements of creatures. Three main stances exist for the feet: weight forward, weight on the rear foot, and weight to the side.

T'ai chi chuan is widely practiced in China and by Chinese living outside of China. Besides being an art form and exercise regime, it is a social activity, especially for the elderly. Early one morning, looking out from my hotel window in Beijing, I saw t'ai chi being practiced in a nearby park. A sea of people in loose jackets moved in unison in a series of graceful movements, like a ballet without music. When I was young my mother would go through a t'ai chi routine at the start of her day.

In the Western world today, t'ai chi is generally used as an exercise. It provides moderate aerobic training, good motor-skill development, training in memory and concentration, moderate muscular strength and endurance, and flexibility training. The movements are largely low impact. The regime provides for the overall well-being of both mind and body. T'ai chi is not, however, geared to specific muscle development or body conditioning, although martial forms of t'ai chi provide for greater development of muscle strength and power.

The Alexander Technique

The Alexander Technique was developed by Frederick Matthias Alexander. He set up the first training school for teachers of the technique in 1931, but practice of the technique dates back to the late 1890s and early 1900s. The Alexander Technique does not involve an exercise program and does not purport to be one. It basically promotes awareness of how we perform our daily activities, and of our posture, balance, and coordination. By becoming aware of our body, we become conscious of the excessive muscular tension within it. This awareness is important because muscular tension is ultimately responsible for poor posture; poor posture, in turn, causes many of the ailments that people ascribe to aging and wear and tear. From awareness, the next step is to reeducate the body to move and stand in improved ways so that equilibrium is restored.

To become free of muscular tension is an important objective of the Alexander Technique. To achieve this, people are prompted to stop and do nothing for a few minutes in order to prevent muscle tension from building up. The exercises prescribed relate mainly to matters of observation. First the practitioner observes herself in a mirror to see how she stands, sits, and moves; the angle of her head; whether one shoulder is up or down; the alignment of her spine; and so on. Second she observes and executes moves without the mirror but while mentally registering them. Finally she checks in the mirror to see if what she perceived as being executed was in fact what she did. For example, if, with her eyes closed, she attempts to stand "correctly," i.e., with a straight back and feet aligned and pointing forward, when she opens her eyes and looks into a mirror, she may find that in reality her feet

are not aligned and her body is turned slightly to one side or the other. After the observation comes the education. To reeducate and bring about an improved way of standing or moving under the Alexander Technique may require doing the very thing that feels wrong. The problem is complicated by the fact that people usually move in the way that they find most comfortable. There is also a need to reeducate response patterns by inhibiting the immediate automatic reaction in order to provide the opportunity for a different, better-informed reaction.

The Alexander Technique gives priority and importance to how the neck is held. When the neck muscles are overly tight, they interfere with the body's movements and throw it out of balance, because the head, which leads the body, is not aligned properly with the spine. The dynamic relationship between the neck and head is referred to as *primary control*. When this is not in balance, our reflexes will not be coordinated. Alexander illustrated the point with the example of a horse. When a rider pulls the horse's head back, the animal loses coordination and comes to a standstill.

The Alexander Technique is not an exercise program in the normal sense of the word. It uses body awareness, improved posture, movements, and coordination to reduce muscle tension, which Frederick Alexander identified as a major cause of many stress-related illnesses, including hypertension, coronary heart disease, gastrointestinal problems, headaches, migraine, insomnia, arthritis, and backache.

Pilates

Pilates is a body-conditioning program founded in the 1920s by Joseph H. Pilates. It focuses on three areas of the body: the abdomen, lower back, and buttocks, which collectively are referred to as the *core*, or *power center*, of the body. Like the Alexander Technique, t'ai chi, and yoga, Pilates promotes body awareness and correct breathing to promote efficient movements, flexibility, and muscle strength. The emphasis in each of these programs is on breathing with the diaphragm. They teach that if we breathe shallowly, the diaphragm fails to flatten out to its fullest capacity. This is in part a result of not exhaling fully, hence, the emphasis in yoga on long exhalation. When the lungs are emptied they can be filled more efficiently. By being aware of a need to create space within the thorax for expansion of the lungs, and by going through the motion of actually creating space during the exercise (what in Pilates is call "zipping up" and "zipping down"), we breathe more effectively and efficiently.

Pilates takes two forms: fitness Pilates and rehabilitation Pilates. The former is for those interested in general fitness, sports training, or postural improvement. The latter is used mainly by people who have been injured and need muscle rehabilitation and is mainly taught one-on-one and using equipment.

Fitness Pilates workouts can be carried out either on mats using body resistance, the most common method, or using apparatus. Apparatus sessions use a wide range of equipment—with names like the reformer, cadillac, wall unit, chairs, pedipull, ladder barrel, and barrels—to provide the resistance required for pushing and pulling activities. Irrespective of whether it is mat-based or apparatus-based, the focus is on correct breathing and body alignment. Pilates has many features in common with yoga and the Alexander Technique. It is primarily a body-conditioning and relaxation program.

Holistic but Not Whole: Aerobics Is the Missing Element

This very quick look at yoga, t'ai chi, the Alexander Technique, and Pilates reveals a common factor: They all emphasize body control via improved breathing and body alignment. Through slow and controlled movement, they allow the mind to become more aware of the body. The focus on breathing and relaxing helps to destress muscles. These programs are holistic in the sense of bringing self-awareness and body movements together. They contrast with physical regimes such as sports, aerobic dance, and other exercise-to-music classes, in which mental awareness is tuned to respond to external forces in a quick and coordinated way. Another way these programs contrast with energetic regimes is in the fact that they promote relaxation *during* the process of self-concentration (or withdrawal), whereas in energetic regimes relaxation *follows* exercise.

As physical regimes, yoga, the Alexander Technique, and Pilates are incomplete. With the exception of t'ai chi, the four practices described in this section provide little aerobic training; that is, they don't do much to raise the heart rate towards the personal maximum. If you breathe slowly, as these programs prescribe, you are bringing the heart rate down. Relaxation is good for the heart, but to build greater strength in the cardiac muscle, few activities equal a good aerobic workout. Hence, these exercises should be used to complement other, more aerobic activities. Finally, all activities carry with them the risk of injuries, and the same applies to these four regimes. Much depends upon how individual instructors school and supervise their students. It is during training to gain the muscle control needed for specific movements that the danger of injury is greatest.

Now let's take an introductory look at combining the best of several methods of exercise.

Finding the Best Combination: The Art and Science of "Fusion" Exercise

Choosing the exercise program that is best for you is entirely personal. For those seeking to incorporate all five fitness components (see Chapter 2 for a review of these) into their workout, one option is to undertake separate sessions of body conditioning, aerobics, stretching, motor-skill development to build muscle strength and endurance, cardiac fitness, flexibility, and coordination. The only problem is the time constraint: There are only seven days in a week! Taking on each component in a rotation would leave little time for anything extra. Besides, doing each component only once a week is not enough, and fitting in more than weekly sessions might be difficult on such a rotation.

For many, combining all the different fitness components into one workout is the best way. Doing so leaves extra time for focusing on priorities. For example, if you get three "complete" workouts, there is still time in your week for extra flexibility training or extra body conditioning. If you are unable to find that extra time, you are at least adequately covered.

To develop an all-encompassing workout, teachers and instructors of fitness should seek to combine the best of all disciplines. The different practices do not have to be mutually exclusive; in fact, as I have shown, they are related. Rather than battling over what method is "right" and "wrong," instructors would be better advised to examine the possibilities offered by the various disciplines.

Aerobic training is essential for the pursuit of a full fitness program. To avoid teaching aerobics because of fears of the possibility of injury is to opt out of the problem. People need to work out aerobically to complement their holistic regimes. The same is true for participants in aerobics, step aerobics, and other exercise-to-music classes. Fears of causing injury have led many to stop recommending certain beneficial positions. Perhaps more time should be spent learning *how* the dangers of getting into certain positions could be eliminated by promoting proper breathing techniques, greater body awareness, and correct body alignment. Certain fundamental principles must of course be observed for safety, but to increase our options and thereby benefit the exerciser—whether that person is ourselves or our student or client—let's examine all the possible angles of our fitness regime. The time has arrived to integrate all that is best into one program.

To this end, in the illustrated exercises presented in the following chapters on body conditioning and flexibility training, I have incorporated the techniques of breathing utilizing the diaphragm and of pelvic- and abdominal-muscle control for achieving core stability. It should be noted that the concept of breathing with the diaphragm is not the invention of sports physiologists; it is simply good practice, based on human anatomy and physiology, as discussed in Chapter 3.

I would also like to stress that I have not adopted these exercises piecemeal. The foundations of many holistic practices lie in antiquity. My approach has been to go back to the drawing board and revisit the musculoskeletal structure, the movements of muscles, the points of insertion and attachment, and the energy systems in order to develop new exercises or to adapt existing ones to make them more effective and safe. By grounding the fusion fitness program in science and by explaining my methods, I hope to move beyond a didacticism that assumes readers will simply follow my recommendations because they're "good for you." (For more details on the concept, science, and philosophy of fusion theory and exercises, see Chapters 8 and 9.)

As sports science evolves and matures, more changes are likely to occur in the theory of how to achieve optimal fitness. This book offers just a beginning—but I hope it is a constructive one. Now let us move on to a discussion of the warm-up.

6

The Warm-Up:
Getting Ready to Exercise

The importance of a warm-up was touched upon in the opening chapter. This chapter considers the benefits of a warm-up in greater detail, addresses what a warm-up should include, and gives examples of how to prepare for different sports activities.

What Is a Warm-Up?

A warm-up is simply the performance of movements that prepare the body for more strenuous activities to follow. It includes movements that mobilize the joints, movements that raise the pulse rate to increase the blood supply to working muscles, and a preparatory stretch.

The preparatory stretch is always done *after* the joints have been mobilized and the pulse rate raised. Whether we mobilize first before raising the pulse rate or vice versa varies with the activity and the environment. In aerobics classes, the mobilizer typically comes before the pulse raiser, but if the room or weather is very cold, it may be better to boost blood circulation first by raising the heartbeat. So some judgement is needed. Moreover, the distinction between the two activities is not always absolute. Activities that raise the pulse rate inevitably involve movement of joints, but they are

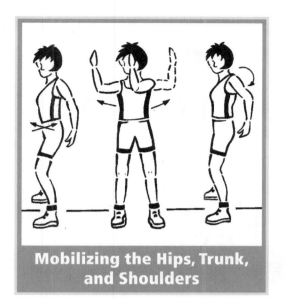

Mobilizing the Hips, Trunk, and Shoulders

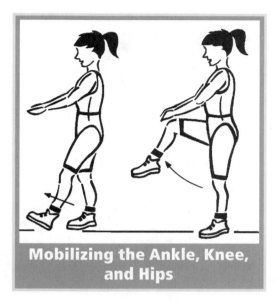

Mobilizing the Ankle, Knee, and Hips

not usually focused on the joints as such. For example, marching briskly, a typical pulse-raising activity, moves the hip joint slightly, but mobilization of the hip joint would involve actions focused specifically on the joint, such as pelvic tilts and rotating the hips with the feet stationary.

Mobilizing the Joints

Muscles can bring about movement only when they cross a movable joint. It follows that if the joints are stiff, any strong muscle movement will cause stress on the joint it crosses and could easily result in injury. The muscles, including the tendons via which they insert into the bones, can also be damaged. Joints need to be introduced gently to the full range of their natural movements before embarking on strenuous activities.

This ensures that the synovial fluid is warm and can act efficiently as both a lubricant and a buffer against impact.

The emphasis given to particular joints depends on the physical activities that follow, as well as those preceding, the exercise. People coming straight from the office, where they have been sitting at a computer, would benefit from more shoulder- and hip-mobilizing moves. These ball-and-socket joints, which are capable of the most diverse movement, are also the most susceptible to injury. The ankle and knee are also highly susceptible, largely because they carry the weight of the body and partly because the attached muscles are of unequal strength. The most important among the list of "musts" for mobilization are the hip, or pelvic, joint, shoulder joint, thoracic and

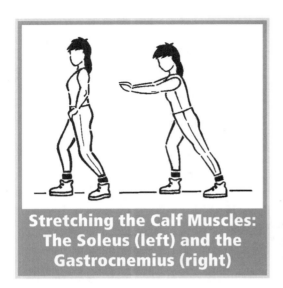

Stretching the Calf Muscles: The Soleus (left) and the Gastrocnemius (right)

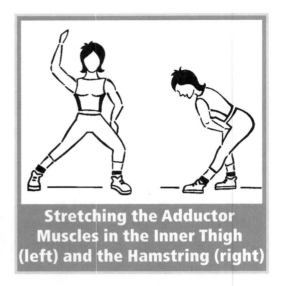

Stretching the Adductor Muscles in the Inner Thigh (left) and the Hamstring (right)

lumbar regions, knees, and ankles (see figures on the previous page), because they usually bear the brunt of most activities. Circling the shoulders, rotating the hips, flexing the ankles, pointing the toes, bending the knees, side bends, and rotating the upper torso with the hips stationary are all examples of mobilizing moves.

Raising the Pulse Rate

The objective in a warm-up is to increase the heartbeat to some 50–60 percent of the personal maximum, in order to increase the blood supply to working muscles and their connective tissues, including tendons and ligaments, so that they are warm and pliable. They will then be ready to take on a greater workload. Rhythmic movements that involve the large muscle groups and that can be slowly increased in intensity—

such as marching/brisk walking, side steps, and step touches—are widely used in aerobics classes. Generally, this part of the warm-up is similar to the main aerobics component, except that it is slower, is much lower in intensity, and excludes explosive movements such as jumps and high kicks. Obviously the approach will vary according to the fitness of the participant. Again, some degree of judgement is needed.

Preparatory Stretches

Stretches should be done only after you are warm, otherwise they can be harmful. For example, if you are a runner or have arrived in the gym for a workout on, say, the treadmill, do not stretch immediately. Take a few minutes first to mobilize joints, loosen up muscles, and increase blood flow. All the muscles that are to be used in activities fol-

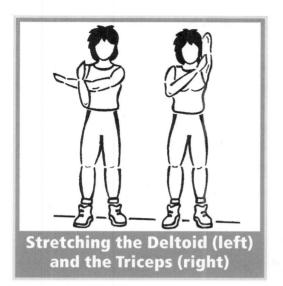

Stretching the Deltoid (left) and the Triceps (right)

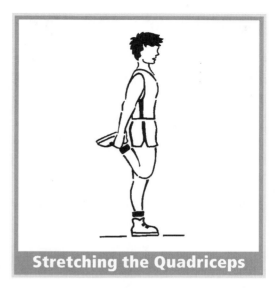

Stretching the Quadriceps

lowing the warm-up must be stretched. Usually this would include the gastrocnemius (the main calf muscles), the soleus (inner calf), the hamstring, and the adductors. These are normally the muscles most used in any exercise regime. Runners would focus on the hamstring, shin, and calves. Rowers would prepare with greater emphasis on the arms (deltoids, biceps, and triceps), trape-zius, pectorals, and quadriceps. Aerobic and body-conditioning classes would also include stretches for the quadriceps, the erector spinae, the lumbar, and the arms (deltoids and triceps).

Generally, in aerobics classes, stretches are performed in a standing position to maintain the raised heartbeat. Pulse-raising movements are also usually made between stretches in order to maintain the heart rate. This helps participants move smoothly into the aerobic component of the class. Sprinters, on the other hand, might do their preparatory stretches on the ground, because the stretch it provides is more intense. Doing a stretch supported by a wall or on the ground often helps in holding the stretch with less pressure on the joints.

Warm-up stretches are usually held for about 10 to 12 seconds, but there is no fixed rule. It can vary with the activity and level of training and flexibility of those involved. Runners often hold stretches for 25 to 30 seconds; by way of contrast, in aerobic classes, this is the length of time recommended for cool-down rather than warm-up stretches. The figures on page 72 and above illustrate some of the main preparatory stretches. More examples of stretches are illustrated in the flexibility training information provided in Chapter 10.

The Benefits of a Warm-Up

Sport research has shown that a warm-up before the main exercise substantially reduces the incidence of sports injuries. By keeping muscles warm and joints well lubricated, warming up reduces muscle tear and damage to joints. The cardiorespiratory system is allowed to build up gradually to the increased demand about to be made on it. This avoids the discomfort, including giddiness, palpitations, and breathlessness, that can be provoked by a sudden increase in exertion. By sending preparatory signals to the brain that warn it of the type and range of activities the body is likely to be undertaking, warming up also improves the body's pattern of response and encourages good-quality movement.

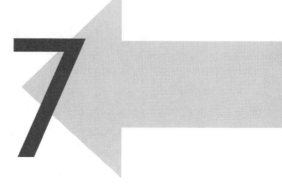

Aerobic Training:
Staying on the Curve

Aerobic activities include all physical exercises that are powered by the oxidation of food through a continuous cycle of ATP synthesis and energy release (see Chapter 3, the section titled "Energy and Energy Systems"). Aerobic activity can be carried out for a sustained period of time when the intensity of the exercise is reasonable. This means an intensity that is sufficient to make the workout effective for improving the cardiovascular and respiratory system, but not so hard that fatigue sets in and/or the anaerobic energy system takes over. Taking all these factors into account, experts recommend a training zone between 60 and 80 percent of the personal maximum heartbeat (see Chapter 2).

One's overall plan for exercise should be based on the FITTA principle, which stands for **F**requency, **I**ntensity, **T**ime, **T**ype, and **A**dherence. Careful planning of these five elements is needed when embarking on an activity, because sporadic exertions bring little benefit. After two weeks of rest or inactivity, some 50 percent of the fitness gained can be lost. Time must be set aside for regular exercise.

Regular aerobic activities contribute, over time, to important physiological changes in the body. Many of these changes relate to the cardiovascular and respiratory systems. The heart increases in size and volume: The left ventricle, in particular, becomes stronger and more effective in pushing oxygenated blood into the aorta and on to the body. Each contraction propels a larger volume of blood than the one before it: Both the stroke volume and maximum cardiac output increase. The improvement in the heart means that it does not work so hard in everyday life. Hence, blood pressure improves both at rest and during activity, and the same exercise routine carried out regularly over a period of time does not require the same effort.

Not only the heart improves: The number of blood capillaries increases in response to the larger volume of blood being handled. Men in training have a capillary density in their muscles as much as 40 percent higher than those who lead a sedentary life. The larger number of capillaries means that the oxygen released in the muscle increases. The body's other internal organs also benefit from the improved blood supply. The lungs become adapted to greater demands for oxygen, and both the tidal volume and the oxygen intake increase. These improvements contribute significantly to reducing or ameliorating coronary heart diseases such as hypertension.

Muscles also benefit from aerobic activities. The muscle fibers change to contain more myoglobin, the oxygen-carrying pigment responsible for oxygen storage and release in muscle cells. Like hemoglobin in red blood cells, myoglobin contains iron

and protein. There is a surge in the number of mitochondria, the tiny structures within the cell that are responsible for energy storage and release.

During training, total body mass and fat are reduced and lean body mass is increased. This helps raise the overall basal metabolic rate. As a result, aerobic activities, especially when complemented by healthy eating, help promote weight control or loss. Overall, someone who exercises regularly will feel and look better.

Programming Effective Training: The Aerobic Curve

Careful planning is required to keep within the aerobic training zone. First, the activity must build up in intensity to reach the training zone. The length of the buildup varies substantially depending on the chosen aerobic activity and personal fitness. It generally takes 2 to 5 minutes for the cardiovascular/respiratory systems to respond to increased physical demand. Discomfort, even cramps, can occur if intense activity is rushed into. People who have not exercised before or who have had a long break from exercise generally need more time for the buildup. More time may also be advisable in a cold environment. Once perspiration begins, the body is ready for more intensive activity,

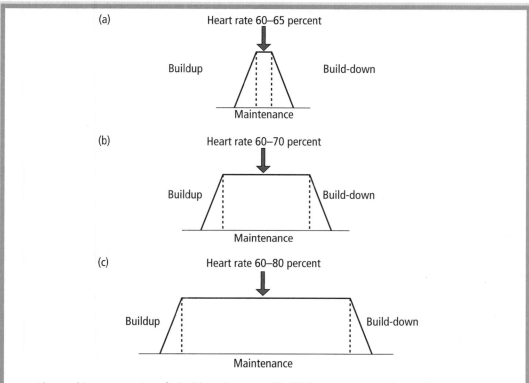

The aerobic curve consists of a buildup, plateau, and build-down. Beginners (a) spend less time in the plateau maintaining the target heart rate than intermediate (b) and advanced students (c). The intensity of exercise increases with training.

Aerobic Training Curves

Effective Personal-training Zones

Age	Personal maximum heart rate	
	60 percent	80 percent
20	120	160
25	117	156
30	114	152
35	111	148
40	108	144
45	105	140
50	102	136
55	99	132
60	96	128

which can be increased until the training zone is reached.

To remain within the plateau of the training zone, the intensity of the workout has to be varied. In a dance or aerobics class, a combination of low- and high-impact moves is used to keep within the zone and to avoid involving the anaerobic energy system. Once the desired level of aerobic training has been attained, the intensity of the movements is gradually reduced. This build-down helps to bring the heartbeat steadily back to its normal rate, and is essential to avoid the pooling of blood in the calf muscles.

Together, the buildup to the training zone, the maintenance of activity at this plateau, and the subsequent build-down constitute the *aerobic curve*. The aerobic curve varies according to the needs and objectives of participants. In a simple aerobic curve, the aim essentially is to work towards a peak heart rate while remaining in the training zone. A fit person requires less time for the buildup and build-down and can spend more time in the training zone. The figure on page 77 provides an example of the proportion of time that could be spent by a beginner and an advanced trainer in the different phases of aerobic training. The table on page 77 provides estimates of the target heart rates within the effective training zone. These decline with age.

Different Kinds of Aerobic Training

Running

A variety of techniques are used in training for running. Hill training sessions, for example, make the leg muscles contract more forcefully than normal. Uphill training increases the concentration of aerobic enzymes in the leg muscles, which eventually adapts the muscles to work at high levels without fatigue. The run could be sequenced as follows: a warm-up jog (equivalent to an aerobic buildup), followed by a fast uphill jog, then a downhill jog to allow some recovery, followed again by an uphill stint. The sequence is repeated four to five times. The number of repetitions varies with a person's fitness, but generally the "reps" should be increased with increased fitness. The uphill run could also be increased and the downhill recovery run reduced in order to increase the intensity of the workout. The sequencing means that several aerobic peaks are involved.

The concept of *fartlek*, meaning "speed play" in Swedish, underlies some of the training methods used by runners. *Fartlek* imitates race conditions, where it is necessary to surge forward to break away from other runners. Here, too, sudden peaking is involved, but the duration of these sequences is not predetermined. For example, the training might involve running until someone on a bicycle is about to overtake the runner, then running faster to try to prevent it, and once having been overtaken, slowing down. Because the runner cannot anticipate when the next bicycle is going to pass her, the spurt does not occur at regular intervals.

Long-distance running involves yet another technique. Training for marathons by regularly running long distances depletes muscle fibers of glycogen and may even damage them because of the repeated accumulation of lactic acid. The general consensus among trainers is that the intensity of training, not the duration, is important. In other words, running slowly for a long distance is less effective as a preparation for a marathon than running fast for a shorter distance. Based on a principle similar to *fartlek*, the recommendation is to inject short spurts of speed every few minutes into the run. This helps to activate the fast-twitch muscles without causing lactic acid to accumulate. Increasing the aerobic potential of fast-twitch muscle fibers helps in a long-distance run when the slow-twitch muscles start to fatigue, generally after about 45 minutes. This form of training is beneficial because it teaches the body to burn fat and conserve glycogen. Here, too, the aerobic curve is multipeaked, but the peaks occur at greater frequency.

Treadmills are useful aids to training because they remove the element of uncertainty in weather and terrain and can imitate uphill, flat, and downhill conditions. Running on the treadmill is obviously different from running outside; it requires less energy for the same speed because the runner is unaffected by the elements, particularly the wind and the unevenness of the ground. Training needs can be simulated to some extent on the treadmill by varying the angle and the speed.

Aerobics and Fitness Classes

Classes involving exercising to music, such as jazzercise, kickboxing, step aerobics, and aerobic dance, are generally considered to be aerobic, although in most cases they also have some anaerobic components. Most of these classes are designed to embrace all five principles of fitness: cardiovascular efficiency, strength, endurance, motor skills, and flexibility. Usually they start with a warm-up, followed by aerobics, body conditioning (muscular strength and endurance), and stretch. Purely aerobics classes, by way of contrast, concentrate primarily on cardiovascular efficiency and generally incorporate little or no body-conditioning or floor work. The following discussion focuses on the aerobic component of exercise-to-music classes and can also be used to design pure aerobic classes.

The most commonly used training structure in aerobic components or classes is a single-peak aerobic curve, wherein participants build up to a peak heart rate, which is maintained for a period according to the fitness of the class or individual. Thereafter the intensity of the exercise is reduced until the heartbeat returns more or less to the starting rate. The buildup begins with rhythmic hand and leg movements that are low in both intensity and impact. These movements are then gradually interspersed with higher impact/higher intensity ones; the tempo of the music rises and the beat becomes more motivating. The alternation of movements continues, all the time increasing the intensity of the exercise, until the ratio of the high-impact/high-intensity moves to low-impact/low-intensity ones is much larger. When the peak is reached, the ratio of high- to low-impact movements might be maintained for a while (see the figure on page 77), after which comes the build-down. Gradually the arm and leg movements are reduced and the music slows. The low-impact/low-intensity moves increase until they are predominant. A double- or multipeak sequencing of aerobic training can also be followed using this pattern.

After deciding on the aerobic structure, the next step is to plan its execution. To do this we draw upon a bank of movements that have been devised for aerobics. Some of the most frequently used ones are illustrated to the right and on subsequent pages. The buildup would start with low-impact moves, which are generally gentler movements that always keep at least one foot on the ground. Examples include the brisk walk, grapevine, step tap, scoops, and box steps. The vigor of these movements can be increased moderately with more intense low-impact moves, such as side and back lunges (extending the leg to side and back), heel digs (flex the foot with the heel on the ground), and low knee lifts. In the case of arms, gentler movements are those with shorter arm leverage, such as biceps curls and the upright row. The higher you raise the arms, the greater the intensity of the workout because the heart has to work harder to pump blood to them. Big staccato

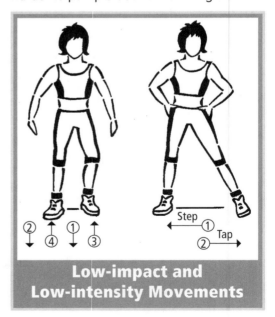

Low-impact and Low-intensity Movements

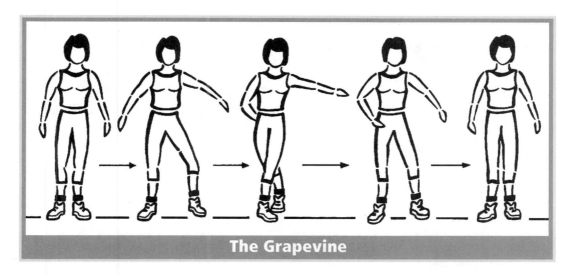

The Grapevine

movements, such as punching, are also more energetic than smooth flowing ones, such as arms swaying from side to side.

As the intensity increases, all the above steps could be executed with a bounce, with one foot still on the ground, initially at low levels and possibly followed by higher foot lifts at increased speed. By this time the point in the curve would probably have been reached where high-impact moves might be incorporated. High-impact is when both feet come off the ground at once and might include jumping jacks, flick kicks, power jumps, power lunges, fast jogs, and knee lifts, accompanied by a jump that brings both feet off the floor.

It is important to alternate high- and low-impact moves to avoid excessive stress on the musculoskeletal structure and possible injury. The high-impact moves encourage an increase in the aerobic capacity of the fast-twitch muscles, thereby increasing endurance when they come to the aid of

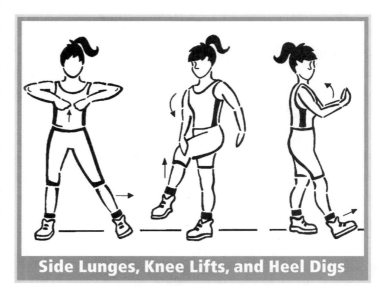

Side Lunges, Knee Lifts, and Heel Digs

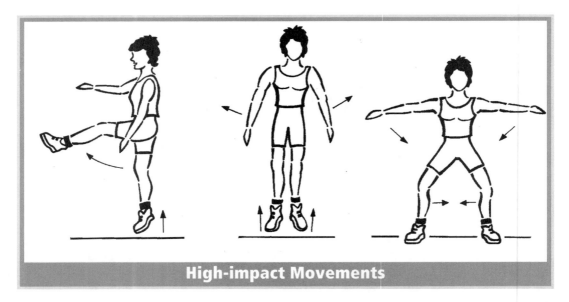

High-impact Movements

fatiguing slow-twitch muscles. This is similar in effect to the training for long-distance running mentioned earlier.

The appropriate mix of low- and high-intensity and -impact movements depends on the age, fitness level, and objectives of the participants. In general, low-impact aerobics are recommended for beginners, overweight individuals, those with a low level of fitness, the elderly, and individuals who have not exercised for a while. For these candidates, the progression along the aerobic curve would involve only low-impact movements. Intensity is increased by a moderate quickening and strengthening of leg and arm movements.

While low-impact aerobics can be used safely throughout the aerobic routine, the same cannot be said for high-impact. Attempting to train aerobically using only high-impact moves would almost certainly lead to exhaustion. Whatever the mix in terms of high- and low-impact, the movements must be varied to give interest. A complete class must ensure that all big muscle groups are worked and all-around training achieved. Excessive repeats can result in boredom, exhaustion, and even injuries, causing the participant to move out of the aerobic curve and the training zone. At the extreme, unbalanced muscular development occurs.

Circuits and Other Aerobic Activities

In a classroom environment, circuits are a popular form of aerobic training. People can do them at their own pace, and thus the training zone can be varied to suit the personal maximum. At the same time, stations

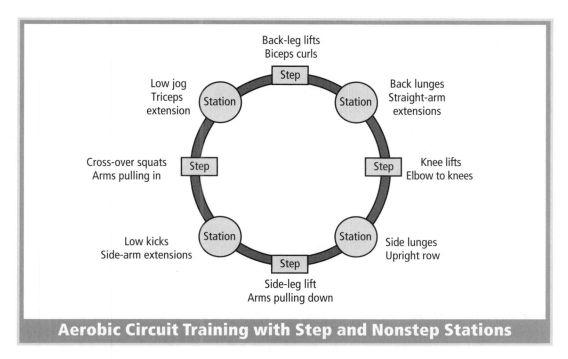

Back-leg lifts
Biceps curls
Step

Low jog
Triceps
extension
Station

Station
Back lunges
Straight-arm
extensions

Cross-over squats
Arms pulling in
Step

Step
Knee lifts
Elbow to knees

Low kicks
Side-arm extensions
Station

Station
Side lunges
Upright row

Step

Side-leg lift
Arms pulling down

Aerobic Circuit Training with Step and Nonstep Stations

in the circuit can be arranged to provide whatever peaking sequence is desired. Circuit training provides variety, reducing any likelihood of muscle overuse. However, to keep this an aerobic activity and to avoid a sudden drop in heart rate, it is inadvisable to have stations such as abdominal crunches following vigorous activities such as lunges, high kicks, and jumping jacks. The sudden switch to a prone position can lead to giddiness and a loss of aerobic efficiency.

Aerobic training using circuits requires at least three minutes at each station using a moderate intensity of exercise. This is the minimum time needed to build up to a sufficiently high oxygen uptake. Up to 12 minutes might be needed at low-intensity levels.

If the same big-muscle groups are used in consecutive stations, the duration at each station should be at the minimum. The increased time that needs to be spent at each station in an aerobic circuit contrasts with the requirements of strength development.

Prolonged resistance training to build up strength of any single muscle group would result in an accumulation of lactic acid and fatigue. Rest intervals are vital for strength training and, since they allow the heartbeat to slow, it is preferable to keep strength training as a separate activity, for example at the end of the aerobic circuit session before the cool-down and stretch. This is not to say that circuits should not be used for muscular strength and endurance training, but aerobic circuits are best kept separate from them.

Many outdoor activities such as walking, cycling, cross-country skiing, rowing, and swimming are also good aerobic activities. As with conventional aerobic training, the principle of alternating the pace of the activities should be applied where feasible.

Avoiding Overtraining

Reference has already been made to the importance of training regularly. While busy people can find this difficult, for others the problem is overzealousness. This can easily lead to overtraining, with harmful rather than beneficial results.

Training is based on the principle of overload, giving the muscles more work than usual. It is, therefore, about physical stress and stimulus on the musculoskeletal system to encourage improvement. If this is overdone regularly, the overtraining syndrome sets in. Instead of maintaining the exhilaration that comes after a good workout because of the healthy dose of endorphins that is released into the system, chronic fatigue sets in and remains throughout the day. Other symptoms include raised heart rate early in the morning, slow recovery of heart rate after training, muscle soreness, absence of menstruation, susceptibility to infection, weight loss, and even diarrhea and intestinal imbalance.

The body, exhausted from the incessant abuse, is giving out important signals that have to be recognized and treated. In the case of an athlete training for competition, these symptoms indicate that he or she has gone beyond his or her peak performance. More training does not necessarily mean better results, because the dividing line between peak performance and overtraining is very fine. For those working out to lose weight, the feeling of sluggishness brought on by overzealous training could easily inspire "comfort" eating.

The overtraining syndrome appears to affect athletes engaged in aerobic activities, especially long-distance runners, more than those involved in anaerobic sports. Anaerobic sports (which rely on lactate as an energy source) provide less opportunity for overtraining, because fatigue sets in quickly, inhibiting further training.

The chronic overtraining syndrome must be treated with complete rest for as long as six weeks, during which time depression may set in because of the enforced inactivity. To avoid overtraining, rest days must be incorporated into the exercise regime to allow muscles and body cells to recuperate. Other forms of milder activities could be undertaken during this period. To restore glycogen levels in the muscles, an interval of some 24 hours between intensive training sessions is required.

8

Body Conditioning: Training for Strength and Endurance

Training for strength and endurance results in significant beneficial changes in the body. The number of muscle fibers increases, as does the proportion of fast-twitch muscles. The net result is an increase in the force and power muscles can exert, as well an extension of the range and type of physical work that can be done. The presence of more muscle fibers increases the lean body mass and with it the basal metabolic rate. Strengthening the postural muscles provides more support to the skeletal frame and helps improve posture and body shape. Strengthening the muscles used in movement improves physical performance generally. Strength training helps individuals whose muscles have atrophied after long illnesses to regain the ability and confidence to move and work. Conditioned muscles look better, perform better, and endure better.

The objectives of training for strength and endurance can go beyond muscle tone. Body builders, for example, train intensively using high external resistance (weights, etc.) to increase muscle bulk. Sprinters and discus and javelin throwers also train for strength. Each of these pursuits benefits from its own particular training regime. This chapter, however, will focus on muscle tone rather than such specialist training regimes.

Basic Principles of Muscle Contraction

Muscles work through contraction in one of three ways (see figure on page 87):

* *concentrically*—the muscle shortens, bringing the two ends closer together

* *eccentrically*—the muscle lengthens under tension to its normal length

* *isometrically* or *statically*—the length of the muscle remains unchanged under tension as the muscle holds a position

In sit-ups or abdominal crunches, for example, the rectus abdominus, which originates from the pubic bone and inserts into the ribs, contracts concentrically, lifting the trunk upward. When the trunk returns to its normal position, the rectus abdominus contracts eccentrically because it is returning to its normal length under tension (see figure on page 88). In squats, the quadriceps contract eccentrically when going down and concentrically when going up. In push-ups, the downward phase involves the eccentric contraction of the pectorals, while the upward phase involves a concentric contraction. In brief, concentric contractions occur when the direction of movement is opposite from the pull of gravity; eccentric contractions occur in the direction of gravity.

Concentric and eccentric contractions come under the heading of *isotonic training*, which aims to allow the muscle to develop tension in opposing movement. In practice, the tension varies depending on the angle of the lever at the joint and the speed of the contraction or movement. In eccentric contraction, the downward phase of the movement, the muscle has to work with gravity and must act as a brake to stop the limb or the body part being moved from falling suddenly. This creates greater resistance for the muscle at work. If the eccentric phase is lengthened by slowing the downward motion, the muscle is put to greater effort and tension. In a progressive training program, therefore, the ratio of concentric and eccentric contractions is varied and their duration of implementation lengthened to provide the overload needed to improve strength.

Static contractions, that is, those allowing the muscle to develop tension without varying the length of the muscle, are used in *isometric training* regimes. Although loosely referred to as static contractions, the prime mover muscle does shorten internally, but because it is offset by a contraction of the antagonist (opposing) muscle, the muscle length appears unchanged. In most cases, these contractions are generally effected by holding a position.

Isometric training is useful when there is insufficient space for sweeping movements. More importantly, it is useful for de-

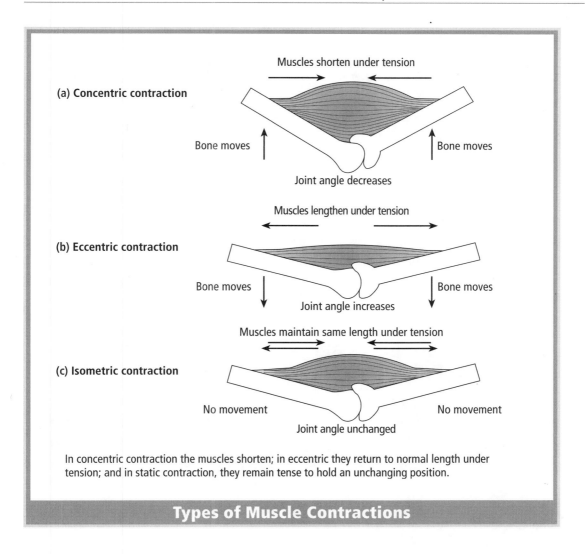

(a) Concentric contraction

Muscles shorten under tension

Bone moves

Bone moves

Joint angle decreases

(b) Eccentric contraction

Muscles lengthen under tension

Bone moves

Bone moves

Joint angle increases

(c) Isometric contraction

Muscles maintain same length under tension

No movement

No movement

Joint angle unchanged

In concentric contraction the muscles shorten; in eccentric they return to normal length under tension; and in static contraction, they remain tense to hold an unchanging position.

Types of Muscle Contractions

veloping strength at specific spots (in the muscle around the joint where it is targeted) for specific activities that require a position to be sustained for a long time. This would include activities such as downhill skiing, gymnastics, t'ai chi, and yoga. Since it involves less motion, isometric training avoids sudden changes in the angle of execution,

reducing the incidence and possibilities of injuries to the joints.

For individuals with problems in their joints, such as the knee, static contractions of muscles, in this instance the quadriceps, offer a good introduction to exercise. These advantages bring with them some disadvantages. The impact of isometric training

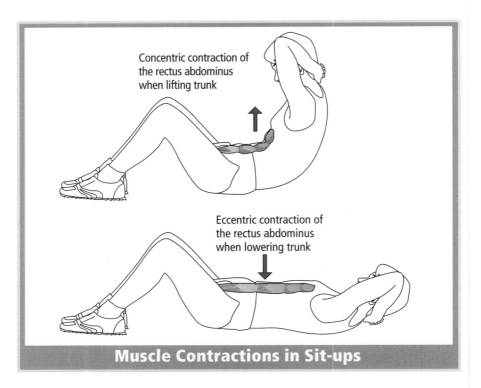

Concentric contraction of the rectus abdominus when lifting trunk

Eccentric contraction of the rectus abdominus when lowering trunk

Muscle Contractions in Sit-ups

is limited to specific target areas. Because isometric contractions do not involve much movement, there is no improvement in motor skills and coordination. Finally, static contractions result in reduced blood flow to the heart during such exertion and higher systolic and diastolic pressures than other strength-training methods.[10] Because of its benefits, isometric exercise has a role to play and remains widely used in the fitness industry, especially with the rise of holistic regimes, and for exercising after injuries. It is important, however, to use isometric training in moderation and in conjunction with isotonic training. It is not recommended for those with heart problems.

Modern technology has focused on these two broad categories of muscle training with the development of equipment that changes the position of the exercise and the speed of contraction and offers different forms of weight to provide added resistance. Faced by a bewildering choice, how should one choose?

Moderation, consistency, and a commitment to the five goals of fitness should, again, serve as the guiding principles. It is important to master the correct techniques and positions for isotonic and isometric contractions using the body as the main resistance before moving on to the use of weights and equipment. If the body is held correctly, it offers an ideal medium, at least initially, for providing the resistance required.

Whether weights are needed depends on the objectives: Do you wish to tone and firm up and maintain this condition, or do you wish to build greater muscle definition or bulk? Although men are more likely than women to build muscle bulk because of the size of their muscle fibers (both slow- and fast-twitch) and greater concentrations of the hormone testosterone, women themselves differ in their propensity to build muscle. Whereas female ectomorphs tend not to build up bulky muscle mass, endomorphs and mesomorphs are more prone to the hypertrophy of muscles (see Chapter 4 for a review of these three basic body types). Therefore, if you fall within the mesomorph or endomorph categories and don't want to increase your muscle bulk, increasing the

number of repetitions might be preferable to increasing resistance by using weights. By contrast, ectomorphs could use weights in a body-building program to increase strength without necessarily building bulky muscles.

Whatever the objectives, good body alignment is necessary for effective and safe strength training. If the body position is incorrectly held, the use of external resistance could exacerbate the injuries that can result. For example, lifting the leg outward and sideways to work the gluteals and the leg abductors (tensor fascia latae) can easily transfer the stress to the small of the back, and if external resistance were to be added through the use of ankle weights, the stress would be even more severe.

It is essential to work opposing muscle groups (see table below). If the quadriceps

Selected Major Opposing-Muscle Groups		
Lower limbs	quadriceps	hamstring
	tibialis anterior	gastrocnemius/soleus
	adductor longus, magnus, and brevis	gluteus medius and minimus, tensor fascia latus
	iliopsoas/hip flexor	gluteus maximus
Upper limbs	flexors of wrists and fingers	extensors of wrists and fingers
	biceps	triceps
	deltoid	latissimus dorsi
Torso	pectoralis	rhomboids/trapezius
	rectus abdominus	erector spinae

are strengthened, for example, the hamstring should be strengthened as well. Otherwise, unbalanced muscle strength will lead to poor posture and unequal stress on the body's musculoskeletal structure. The most widespread example is the problem of shin splints—a fine stress fracture that results in pain at the front and sides of the lower leg. This is common among runners because of the imbalance between their strong gastrocnemius and soleus muscles (the calves) and their weak tibialis anterior muscles (in the shin). An excessive amount of jumping, skipping, and similar high-impact moves in class exercises can also result in shin splints because the powerful contractions of the calf muscles result in their overdevelopment. The gastrocnemius and soleus become tight, causing stress in the opposing muscle, the tibialis anterior. The buildup of pressure in the muscle, a condition known as *compartment syndrome*, causes pain.

The FITTA (frequency, intensity, time, type, and adherence) principle described in the chapter on aerobic training applies also in training for endurance, strength, and body conditioning. While the training should be regular and sufficiently frequent to have an impact (three to four times a week), there must be sufficient rest between training sessions and between muscles worked. The intensity of the training has to be moderated to ensure that muscles are overloaded but not excessively so. Overvigorous training can injure muscle attachments and joints because muscles respond to training much faster than the ligaments and tendons to which they are attached. If intensity is excessive, fatigue sets in, resulting in poor performance, incorrect positions, and injuries.

The type of exercise and the time devoted to it also need careful planning, taking into account objectives, fitness, and age. It is important to stay with an exercise regime and to acquire correct techniques in terms of body alignment and breathing. Switching from one type of strength and endurance training to another will not serve much purpose. To achieve the desired results, consistency is required. Progress can take the form of increasing the resistance, increasing the repetitions, varying the speed of contractions, increasing the duration of the workout, and shortening the rests between the different sets of exercise.

Training Using Body Resistance: The Fusion Recipe

In Chapter 5, I reviewed the various "holistic" regimes—including yoga, t'ai chi, Pilates, and the Alexander Technique—that have grown in popularity in recent years. A common theme runs through all of these; namely, they are popular partly because of the search for safer methods of exercise and the desire by many people for greater tranquillity. We also saw, however, that in practice, not all that is called "holistic" (and here we use the word loosely, because they are not holistic in the sense of being complete fitness programs) is necessarily safe.

Nevertheless, all of these regimes offer elements that are especially beneficial for achieving health and fitness. Benefits include the emphasis on correct body alignment, an awareness of breathing and its use to promote relaxation, and greater stability and control of the body. I have integrated those aspects of the Eastern arts that enhance the tranquillity and safety of workouts into the mainstream exercise regimes of the West. This, however, is not the complete story. In developing the fusion recipe I have also reviewed other practices, such as callanetics and Lotte Berk's methods. They, too, have had an influence on the exercises outlined in the following chapters, so although you will find similarities between the fusion recipe and all the practices mentioned, you will also see significant differences, in terms of both concept and practice.

Correct Body Alignment

The emphasis placed by fusion exercises on body alignment is aimed at bringing mainstream Western exercises in line with some of the more attractive aspects of Eastern practices. This is not to say that Western sports science does not know about body alignment, but knowing and implementing it are two different things. Haste and the tendency in modern life to "get on with it" often mean that people rush to undertake an exercise movement without taking the time to assume the correct body posture. Rarely in the past did body-conditioning classes spend time on aligning the body or getting into the correct starting position. In the fusion recipe for fitness and health, alignment of the body and breathing techniques are the cornerstone of any movements. The focus is to get the body into an alignment where the normal curvature of the spine is maintained (see Chapter 3) without the rigid tensing of the muscular system to hold the body in that position.

It is important to note that this does not necessarily mean a perfectly upright posture with shoulders back, neck stiff, and chin forward, such as is generally associated with, say, a soldier standing at attention or even the rigid stance that we were made to adopt in PE classes when I was a young girl. "Normal" actually means the ability to maintain balance in the body, with the head relaxed on top of the neck, neither too far forward or back, so that the rest of the body does not need to compensate for any potential imbalance. Here I am influenced by the Alexander Technique of body awareness, but taking it well beyond day-to-day activities into the arena of exercise regimes.

In the fusion approach every exercise starts by checking the posture and position of the body. Starting without ensuring that your body is correctly aligned can lead to injuries; conversely, spending a little time to get into the proper alignment optimizes the results you can obtain from the exercises.

You should ensure that your weight is evenly distributed, that you are not standing more on one leg than the other, nor leaning too far forward or backward. Check also that your neck is relaxed and free, that the head sits comfortably on it, and that the shoulders are relaxed, with the shoulder blades down and not rounded forward. The crown of the head should be aligned with the feet; if the head is too far forward, the buttocks will be pushed back to maintain balance, and vice versa. Above all, ensure that the hip, or pelvic area, is wide and stable, and that the back is not rounded or the small of the back pushed forward and the buttocks back. This applies equally whether you are standing, kneeling, or lying on your back. Think of your spine as building blocks stacked on top of each other, perfectly balanced without the need to be held rigidly in place by muscles.

When you are lying on your back, check that you are not slanted or rolled over to one side or the other, that both shoulders are on the floor, and that the weight of the body is evenly distributed with both sides of the buttocks resting evenly on the floor. Your neck should be long at the back; if the head is tilted up, the neck hyperextends and movements can result in stress to the back of the neck. Test to see if you have the correct position by gently raising your head, using both hands to support the base of the skull, and then bringing the chin slightly in toward the chest, freeing the neck. Then gently place the head down again and turn it gently from side to side. You should be able to turn from side to side freely. With practice, you will assume the correct position automatically.

If you are lying on your side, make sure that your legs are stacked on top of each other and that your hip joints are also aligned on top of each other.

If you are on all fours, ensure that the weight of the body is evenly distributed. Check to see if you are pressing more on one hand than the other; check that the hip joint is aligned above the knees; and check also that the back is in a neutral position and not sagging.

Core Stability

When you begin an exercise movement, several things happen. As I have explained in earlier chapters, the main muscle moves to effect the workout (prime mover or agonist muscle), the supporting muscle works to assist the movement (antagonist muscle), and other muscles contract to stabilize the joints (synergist muscles), ensuring that the

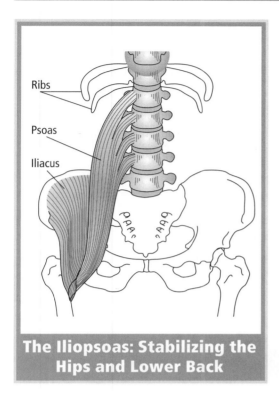

The Iliopsoas: Stabilizing the Hips and Lower Back

Consider performing sit-ups the old-fashioned way, with the legs extended straight in front. This unstable position causes the *iliopsoas* muscle (see figure on the left) to contract synergistically to stabilize the lower trunk, pulling the lower back off the floor, which in turn results in injury and stress to the back. This is a good example of an exercise gone wrong because the stability of the body was not ensured at the outset. How can we ensure stability of the body so as to allow the strengthening of the intended muscle group freely, effectively, and safely?

principal movements are made efficiently and effectively. Without the coordinated and synchronized movements of the synergist muscles, the workout would not be effective and, even worse, injuries could occur. When you pull one limb of a puppet, all the other bits of the body start moving around because there is nothing to make it stable. The human body does not do that, because our muscles automatically act synergistically to stabilize the body during movement. Even so, the body works better if you get into a "correct" body position that facilitates this stabilization.

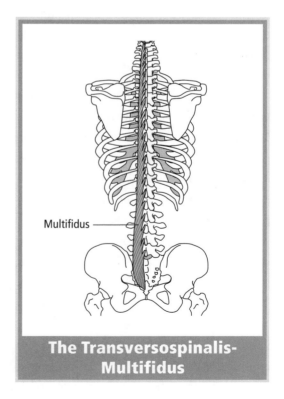

The Transversospinalis-Multifidus

Stability means control. Several key muscles need to be involved in achieving core stability. Among the most important is the transverse abdominus (see page 103). Others include the iliopsoas (which consists of two muscles, the *iliacus* and the *psoas*), the *multifidus* (see figure at the bottom of page 93), the pelvic-floor muscles, the *adductor brevis*, the *rectus abdominus*, the *obliques*, the diaphragm, and the *erector spinae* (see also Chapter 9).

The most important muscle in achieving core stability is the transverse abdominal muscle, because it acts as a corset for the trunk, holding it in position so that the limbs can move from a stable base without distortion or injury to the body, principally protecting the spine and the hip. Engaging the iliopsoas or hip flexor provides stability whenever movements involve the lower limbs or trunk. As explained earlier (see Chapter 5), this is very much in line with the principles of t'ai chi, in which the tan tien (the point three fingers' width below the navel) is regarded as the central core of the body and limb movements as mere extensions of it. In all probability, when t'ai chi originated in ancient China, little was known of muscle structure, hence the use of the mystical description tan tien (heavenly gate) for that part of the anatomy which is vital for core stability. If you stabilize the central core of your body, you move and perform better. This is the principle from which fusion exercises take their cue.

How do we engage these stabilizing muscles? As in most of the Eastern martial practices, including t'ai chi, fusion exercises focus on breathing techniques to engage the transverse abdominal muscles as a stabilizing force (see Chapter 9). You will see over and over again in my descriptions of movements in the following chapters the instruction to inhale while letting the belly expand and, more importantly, to exhale while letting the navel move toward the spine. When breathing out to draw the navel toward the spine, think of an imaginary point lying three fingers' width below the navel and aim to draw that point and the abdominal area below it inward. This engages the transverse abdominal muscles more effectively and allows the rib cage to remain wide and stable for normal breathing. If you allow the navel to move toward the spine when breathing out, but at the same time constrict the upper abdominal muscles, breathing is hampered and the transverse abdominal muscles are not effectively engaged. As you breathe out, sending the navel toward the spine, the diaphragm relaxes and draws with it the transverse abdominal muscles because the two are interconnected. This exhalation creates a hollowing of the abdomen. Almost simultaneously the iliopsoas is also engaged, as the pelvis tilts gently forward to help stabilize the pelvic girdle. This, in turn, stabilizes the trunk and spine as well as the lower limbs. This series of stabilizing movements, initiated by breathing, provides the stable base from which to work.

You can increase stability even more, if need be, by drawing the adductor brevis—the short inner thigh muscles spanning the front part of the pubic and lower hip bone and the femur at the top end of the thigh—inward as though you were doing a pelvic-floor exercise (for more, see the following chapter and especially page 110). This is the key to the breathing techniques used in qi gong for the regulation of energy flow. I have also incorporated this move into the fusion exercises for stretching and relaxation, as you will see in Chapter 10. It is especially beneficial when breathing exercises for relaxation are carried out from a sitting position (normally cross-legged or in half or full lotus), because it provides greater anchorage to the ground, freeing the lungs to respond to the calming effect of the breathing exercise. An additional bonus, of course, is the beneficial impact on the pelvic floor.

My mother used to draw heavily on breathing technique as an expert markswoman. I recall when I was a child that she would spend hours standing in position gripping a hand weight and breathing into the position to stabilize her aim for shooting. My brothers and I often tried in vain to push her. So proud was she of her stability that well into her 60s she was still able to challenge her grandchildren to dislodge her from her stance. It certainly brought its rewards. Among her many achievements, she was a gold medallist in the Asian Festival of Sports of 1975. Now in her 70s, she remains a staunch proponent of t'ai chi and qi gong exercises.

Other muscles can be brought into play to stabilize the body. If the exercise involves the upper limbs, the trapezius can be engaged for this purpose. Arm exercises with rigidly held shoulders are likely to transfer the stress to the neck and the rhomboids—the muscle in the middle of the upper back along the spinal column. By contrast, breathing in to raise the shoulder blade (scapula) and exhaling to bring it down will engage the trapezius muscles to stabilize the upper back, returning the scapula to its normal alignment. This allows the arms to work freely. Exercises involving the lower limbs hinge primarily on the stability of the core pelvic girdle, as described previously, and the alignment of the knee over the ankle.

In all the exercises described in the chapters that follow, I place great emphasis on maintaining normal spinal curvature during the execution of the exercise, in order to avoid stress on the small of the back. In some exercises, however, the starting position might not involve this "neutral" curvature. When lying down on the back, a

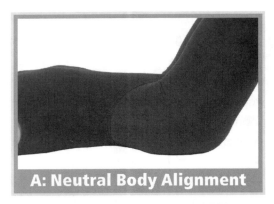

A: Neutral Body Alignment

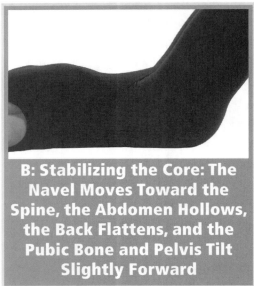

B: Stabilizing the Core: The Navel Moves Toward the Spine, the Abdomen Hollows, the Back Flattens, and the Pubic Bone and Pelvis Tilt Slightly Forward

tion of a small pelvic tilt at the start of the exercise enhances the stability of the pelvic girdle, especially in exercises for the buttock and upper thigh muscles. This increases the effectiveness of the exercise, providing greater resistance to the workout.

While the tilt flattens the lower back slightly at the start of the exercise, normal curvature is resumed once movement commences, leaving the stabilizing muscles to maintain control of the position. In this, fusion exercises converge with the Oriental martial technique of maintaining a stable stance, rather than more modern practices such as Pilates, which starts with a neutral spinal curvature (see sidebar on page 97 for more about how fusion fitness differs from Pilates).

The benefits of maintaining a stable base during movement are significant. Working with a stable base reduces the likelihood of injury, including stress on joints, and especially injury to the back. It improves the performance and effectiveness of the workout because it reduces the involvement of other supporting muscles, allowing the workload of the exercise to fall squarely on the muscle that is being targeted. For example, in raising the leg sideways with a stable base, you are using the outer thigh and buttock muscles (abductors and gluteals) and not the hips (iliopsoas). Significant improvement in posture and bearing will result. Appearance and confi-

normal spinal curvature generally means that the small of the back is raised slightly off the floor, and this position fails to sustain and support the back when the legs are moved, even if the transverse abdominal muscle is engaged. This is especially the case when the stomach muscles are too weak to maintain that so-called corset control. To provide additional support, a very slight pelvic tilt is introduced. The introduc-

dence will improve, and, more importantly, problems generally associated with poor posture, such as back pain, headaches, and poor breathing and movements, will diminish. Engagement of the transverse abdominal muscle will also contribute significantly to a flatter tummy.

Getting It Together the Fusion Fitness Way

Along with studying and adapting the Eastern techniques related to breath control, body alignment, and core stability, I reviewed the musculoskeletal structure and mechanics of the human body. Using the

How Does Fusion Fitness Differ from Pilates?

Because both disciplines emphasize core stability, I have often been asked to explain the difference between the two. The many versions of Pilates make a direct comparison difficult, but the following points are, I believe, relevant in any discussion of fusion fitness and Pilates.

In a typical fusion fitness class, cardiovascular exercises (focused on improving the heart, lungs, and the respiratory and blood circulatory systems) and motor-skill development remain essential components, alongside strength, endurance, and flexibility training. Mat-based Pilates, by contrast, incorporates little or no cardiovascular component or dynamic motor-skill development. Both disciplines place great emphasis on core stability and on the role of the transverse abdominal muscles in providing it, but fusion exercises make greater use of the pelvic roll to maintain core stability. As explained in this chapter, the involvement of the iliopsoas is particularly beneficial when the abdominal muscles are too weak to maintain the core position unaided. In addition, Pilates exercises start with a neutral spinal curvature, while the emphasis in fusion exercise is on maintaining normal spinal curvature during movements.

The portfolio of exercises used in fusion fitness classes is generally different from that used in Pilates, although as in all disciplines there are some similarities. In strength and endurance training, fusion exercises rely on the principle of overload based on a progressive buildup of body resistance to the workout as the participant gains in strength. Both isotonic and isometric training techniques are used, but with a greater emphasis on isotonic exercises. Fusion exercises also have little in common with apparatus-based Pilates.

In structure, fusion classes remain essentially the same as those taught in other exercise-to-music classes. The principle of pursuing all five fitness components remains intact. The fusion recipe, however, brings together all the features that make the holistic regimes effective and sought after and incorporates them within the mainstream of exercise classes while avoiding those movements and positions that are less safe.

I have pursued a "fusion" approach largely because I see little purpose in compartmentalizing the good features of any particular regime, obliging participants to attend separate sessions of different disciplines. Time is precious, and the full panoply of exercise regimes may be unavailable for some individuals. Integration should be the aim, so that the widest possible range of participants can draw upon the best of Oriental and Occidental fitness regimes within a single session.

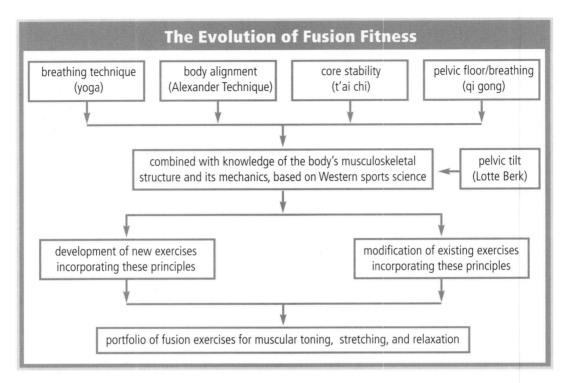

The Evolution of Fusion Fitness

principles of isotonic and isometric contractions, I drew up a series of exercises that would condition the muscles and improve their strength and performance and, in the process, improve the appearance of the body. I drew upon the existing bank of exercises, modifying them in accordance with the principles outlined above. Using this fusion recipe I also developed new exercises to address some of men's and women's specific problem areas.

The following chapters aim to tackle the common problems of flabby tummies, legs, and underarms, love handles, and sagging bottoms. I have achieved considerable success with my own students, who range in age from their late teens to more than 70. Based on my experience, then, permit me to reemphasize a central point of this chapter: It is vital to acquire the techniques of body alignment, breathing, and stability control before rushing to perform these exercises. Spend time acquiring these techniques by stopping when you lose control over body alignment, adjusting your position, and then starting again. With patience, you will find the effort well worth the time. Enjoy the results.

Fusion Exercises: Putting Theory into Practice

In this chapter, I devote a section to each principal muscle group. First I describe the muscles contained in the group, then I describe step-by-step exercises for increasing the various muscles' strength and endurance. The exercises include ones that I have developed and used in my classes after considerable research, practice, and observation of the results. I have also adapted existing techniques to make them safer and more effective, in the process reviving ones that although once popular were deemed potentially unsafe. In doing these exercises, care should be taken to start in the correct position and to breathe properly.

At the start of a training program, when some muscles are weak, stronger ones tend to take over, causing the exerciser to adjust his or her position in order to accommodate this imbalance. In doing so, the exerciser is likely to lose the correct body alignment. If at any point you feel you are losing the correct position, stop, rest, and begin again. It is more important to master the technique than to exercise immediately and intensely but incorrectly. Poor habits are difficult to correct.

I have developed sequences for getting into the correct position for each exercise. I have repeated them throughout the text for easy reference, but once mastered they should automatically become part of what you do.

Even when practicing on my own, I go through the sequence for getting the body into position.

The same principle applies also to breathing. In general, to get into position you exhale while tucking the tummy in (think of the navel moving toward the back of the spine). Thereafter, breathe normally. Also, in general, you breathe *out* while exerting effort—that is, during the contraction of a muscle, e.g., lifting the leg off the floor, raising the trunk in an abdominal crunch, squeezing the knees together, bending the knees, or lowering the trunk in a squat. Likewise, you breathe *in* while releasing the contraction—e.g., as you lower the leg after lifting it. Breathing out as you exert effort allows the central core of the body to remain stable and in correct alignment. Specifically, as explained in Chapter 8 and further elaborated in the section on abdominal muscles that follows, exhaling allows you to engage the transverse abdominal muscle, the body's so-called corset. Conversely, you inhale to refuel your energy and to release the muscle.

This breathing technique is especially important in strong exertions, such as lifting a heavy weight, and in workouts that require high intensity and low reps. However, in many low- to moderate-intensity exercises, in which the objective is both to tone muscle and to build up endurance (as in most floor work in aerobics classes), breath-ing out during moderate exertion of effort is important but probably less critical than maintaining a breathing rhythm that ensures a good and regular supply of oxygen. Once you start with correct body alignment, the chance of going out of alignment during low to moderate exertion is less than in strong exertion. In some exercise sequences where you work both eccentrically and concentrically—for example, when you lift for a count of two and go down for two, or lift for one and go down for three—it might not always be possible to apply this blanket approach of breathing out during exertion. If such a blanket approach were to be adopted, the resulting breathing would be rapid and shallow. Therefore, although I have added reminders to breathe out as you lift and to breathe in as you lower in the exercises that follow (appropriate because they all follow the simple format of lift for one and down for one), once you change to more complex formats of contractions at varying speed, the better solution is to breathe normally. To ensure continued good posture, check the body alignment frequently, stopping whenever you feel that you are moving out of position. Resume the exercise when you feel rested.

Irrespective of the intensity of the exertion, it is essential to breathe correctly when getting into position at the start of the exercise in order to stabilize the central core of the body. It is also useful to remember that although this book places great emphasis on breathing, the technique described is perfectly natural; the practice of breathing with the diaphragm is not a new invention. So do not stress out over the breathing instructions that follow, but above all **do not hold your breath**. Once you have mastered the basic principles mentioned above, the sequence of breathing during the exercise will come naturally.

To build up endurance, repeat each movement until the muscles are working slightly beyond their normal capacity (see Chapter 2 on the principle of overload). There will be a slight accumulation of lactic acid, but as muscles become conditioned they will be able to do more due to an increase in the oxidative capacity of both fast- and slow-twitch muscles and a greater tolerance to lactic acid. To build up strength, increase the body resistance by varying the contraction; for example, by increasing the ratio of eccentric to concentric contractions. In squats, this could mean going down for a count of three and then coming up for a count of one.

I have avoided specifying the number of reps for the exercises. The number will vary with the age and level of fitness of participants, the objective of the class, the way in which the different exercises are sequenced, and even the speed of the music. The slower the music, the harder one must work when training for strength development. Instruc-

tors and exercisers must use their discretion. In a class situation the participant must also rely on his/her own judgement and take a rest when needed. In a mixed-ability class—and most classes fall into this category—it is almost impossible to incorporate the right number of reps for everyone, so instructors should advise class participants to rest whenever they feel tired, and to resume exercising when they feel ready.

In a class where participants are of the same ability, a safe rule of thumb for beginners is to start with one set of 8 reps, and to build from there. For those who are very strong, 4 sets of 8 reps, or slightly more, could be attempted. There is no hard-and-fast rule, except that the participant should aim for an overload, but should not work through pain.

In describing the exercises, I suggest variations. With experience, you will probably be able to devise even more variations. Apply the FITTA principle to progress even further when you are strong enough to do so. Increase the number of reps or the number of sets of each movement. Increase the intensity of the movements—do this by working more slowly, pausing at each movement; increasing the ratio of eccentric to concentric contractions; reducing the rest period between sets of exercise; and increasing the time spent on the exercise.

I have provided a variety of exercises for each muscle to give a choice of options and positions. Although the exercises within each section cater to the same muscle group, they vary in their impact on the different muscles within the group. Avoid performing all of them in one session, however, because doing so would probably be too much, risking strain and possibly injury. Appendix 3 provides examples of training programs that you might find useful.

Music helps keep you going, so if there's music available, turn it on. Choose music that has slow, controlled beats; the slower the music, the harder the workout.

Lower Torso and Legs

The Abdominal Muscles

There are four abdominal muscles: the rectus abdominus, transverse abdominus, obliquus externus (external obliques), and obliquus internus (internal obliques).

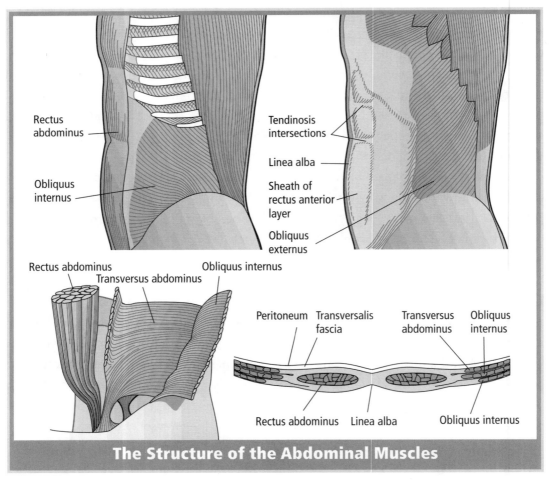

The Structure of the Abdominal Muscles

The *rectus abdominus* is a long strip of muscle that originates from the pubic bone and inserts into the fifth, sixth, and seventh ribs and the *xiphoid process* (the lower end of the sternum). This muscle, broader at the top and narrower towards the pubic end, is divided by the *linea alba*. Contracting, it lifts the upper torso.

The *external obliques* are the largest muscles running on each side of the body from the eight lower ribs down in an oblique line to the iliac crest. The *internal obliques* lie largely beneath this, but they are attached to the iliac crest and run obliquely upward. The uppermost fibers insert into the seventh to ninth costal cartilages, but the lower fibers are joined with the aponeurosis of the transverse abdominus to the pubic crest. (An *aponeurosis* is a sheet of tough, fibrous tissue that acts like a tendon, attaching muscle to the bone.)

The *transverse abdominus*, the innermost stomach muscle, arises at the fascia in the lumbar region of the spine (between the iliac crest and the twelfth rib) and the lower six intercostal cartilages, where it interdigitates (interlocks) with the diaphragm. The transverse abdominus runs transversely, like a corset for the body, one part blending with the internal obliques to insert into the pubic crest and the rest passing into the rectus abdominus.

The Conventional Body Crunch

The most common method of exercising the abdominal muscles is the crunch. This primarily works the rectus abdominus.

- Lie on your back with knees bent and feet hip distance apart. Place your hands on each side of the head, with elbows out wide.

- Using the tummy muscles, raise the trunk off the floor by no more than 30 degrees, and then lower again. Breathe out as you come up, and breathe in as you go down. You should feel a tension in the abdominal muscle, stretching from below the sternum and downward. Be careful not to push the stomach muscles out when raising the trunk.

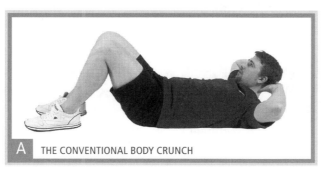

A   THE CONVENTIONAL BODY CRUNCH

- Repeat the movement. The number of repetitions will vary with the individual; you could start with a set of eight and work upward over time to as many as can be sustained.

- Variations in the speed and sequencing of the contractions, such as going up for two counts and down for two, could be introduced to intensify the workout.

The upward movement is a concentric contraction, with the rectus abdominus shortening. It is this shortening that pulls the trunk up. In the downward phase the contraction is eccentric, with the rectus abdominus returning to its normal length under tension. Keep your eyes directed at an angle of about 45 degrees toward the ceiling. A gap should be maintained between the chin and neck, but there should not be any stress on the neck. Do not let the head hang back; give it good support with the hands. It is important to use the hands only for support; they should not be used to pull or jerk the head forward—a common error made when doing this exercise. An alternative position for beginners is to fold the arms across the chest and look down the length of the body when crunching up. In this position, the neck supports the head and the tendency to jerk the head forward is avoided. A disadvantage is the potential for neck ache, because the neck muscles are contracting isometrically to hold the position.

So far I have illustrated the conventional crunch in the manner in which it is normally taught. This exercise can be made safer using the fusion approach to stabilize the core area (abdomen, hips, and lower back). Before raising the trunk, exhale to let the navel move toward the spine and the spine move toward the floor. All the other steps described above remain the same. Note that the extent to which exhaling allows the small of the back to rest on the floor depends on the spinal curvature of the individual. In most cases, with a normal spinal curvature, this exhalation process brings the small of the back in contact with the floor. If the small of the back is still off the floor, it may be more comfortable to place a small towel, folded flat, under the small of the back. The towel is not to hold up the back so that the abnormal curvature is maintained, but to support it after exhalation. I have repeated this recommendation in the following exercises as a reminder.

The body crunch mainly works the rectus abdominus, which is important as an opposing muscle group to the spinal muscles (erector spinae); a strong rectus abdominus can therefore contribute to better posture. Intense training of this muscle will develop a "six-pack"—well-developed ridges of muscles running down from below the chest to the pubis.

Moving Beyond Conventional Crunches

For women, the problem of bulging and flabby tummy muscles is often different from that of men. The uterus lies in front of the digestive system. Normally relatively small, it increases in size during the menstrual cycle and, of course, in pregnancy. The increase is so great in pregnancy that the linea alba, the narrow gap that runs between the two vertical columns of the rectus abdominus, separates, creating a space between the two ridges of the muscle.

The transverse abdominus, the abdominal muscle that acts as a corset to hold the internal organs back, also loosens during pregnancy. Firming this muscle puts the body's natural corset back into its place. Sadly, the muscle is neglected in conventional body crunches. In fact, most people doing conventional body crunches push the stomach muscle out as they strain to raise the trunk, and breathe in instead of out during the process. This does little for the transverse abdominus, although the rectus abdominus is being worked. The result can be a strong overlay of rectus abdominus muscles over bulgy lower tummy muscles, which are difficult to get rid of once developed.

In response to this problem I have developed two exercises, which I call the *transverse* and *reverse abdominal squeezes*. I place great emphasis on breathing with the diaphragm to work these muscles; this is because the transverse abdominus, the innermost abdominal muscle, interdigitates with the diaphragm, and assists in expelling air out of the lungs.

Transverse Abdominal Squeeze

- Lie on your back, with the feet firmly placed hip distance apart, just as for the body crunch.

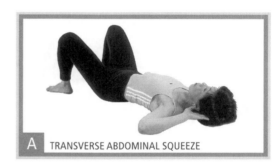

A TRANSVERSE ABDOMINAL SQUEEZE

- Take a deep breath and exhale fully, letting the navel sink towards the spine and letting the small of the back sink toward the floor. Your transverse abdominus should now be engaged. Individuals who suffer from lordosis (an abnormally curved spine) could place a towel, folded flat, under the small of the back, if the back remains off the floor.

- You can work from this position, or, if you are an advanced student, on the

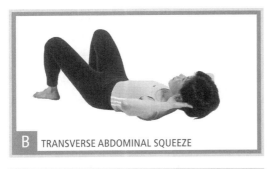

B TRANSVERSE ABDOMINAL SQUEEZE

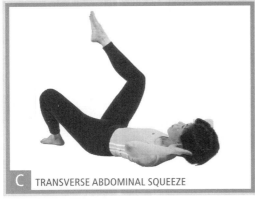

C TRANSVERSE ABDOMINAL SQUEEZE

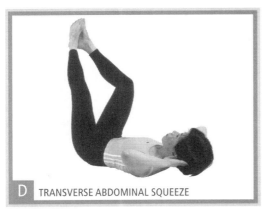

D TRANSVERSE ABDOMINAL SQUEEZE

other foot, also turning the knee outward. Bring the heels together. You now have both legs raised with the knees out and heels together, a bit like a frog. Do not try to raise both feet at the same time because you could lose the muscle tension developed when engaging the transverse abdominus. Remember, your aim is to work the deepest layer of the abdominal muscle.

- With the heels together, squeeze the knees in to touch each other. As you squeeze the knees together, breathe out and tuck in the navel further. You will feel a tightening or contraction of the lower abdominal muscles—your "corset."

- While breathing in, release and let the knees fall apart; the heels should remain together. Repeat, squeezing the knees in and then releasing, until you feel an overload. The performance should be slow and controlled, with even breathing.

Once the technique is mastered you can increase the intensity of the workout and work the surrounding muscles. You can do this, for example, by moving on to the reverse abdominal squeeze, outlined below, without any break between the two exercises. If doing that proves to be too much, rest and start afresh with the reverse abdominal squeeze as a separate exercise.

next out-breath raise both shoulders off the floor while supporting the head with hands on either side of it.

C
D
- Breathing normally, lift one foot, turning the knee outward, and then lift the

Reverse Abdominal Squeeze

This exercise works both the rectus abdominus and the transverse abdominus.

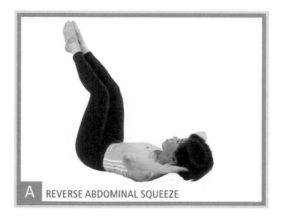

A   REVERSE ABDOMINAL SQUEEZE

- Start from the same floor position as for the transverse abdominal squeeze, with legs bent and feet off the floor.

- This time, once you have brought the knees together, keep them in this position and contract, breathing out and letting the navel sink in as you do so. You will feel a tightening or contraction of the lower abdominal muscles. The pubic bone tilts up slightly and the bent knees move in slightly towards the chest as a result of the contraction of the rectus abdominus.

- Release the contraction and breathe in, letting the navel resume its original position. The release will move the knees slightly away from the torso, allowing them to return to their original position.

- Repeat for as many reps as is comfortable. Add variation by contracting for two counts and releasing for two.

In this exercise, the rectus abdominus muscles near the pubic bone are working actively. This is in contrast to the conventional body crunch, in which the upper torso is raised, causing the upper part of the rectus abdominus to move and the lower part (the point of origin) to remain still. This dif-ference in movement highlights the debate that exists regarding the points of origin and insertion of the rectus abdominus. In pelvic tilts and the reverse abdominal squeeze, the pubic bone is actually moving and the more stable point is where the rectus abdominus attaches to the ribs. As a result, some books identify the ribs as the point of origin for the rectus abdominus, which differs from the more traditional definition of the pubis as the point of origin. In this exercise the iliopsoas muscle works as a synergist to keep the position of the pelvis/hip stable.

Because the movements of the knee and pubic bone are very small, controlled, and, more importantly, a consequence of the abdominal contraction, I describe the exercise as a "squeeze." This distinguishes it from the conventional reverse curl, in which the knees are brought in towards the chest and the hips are lifted up. It is called a *reverse curl* because it is an opposite movement from the trunk curling upward in the conventional crunch. The traditional reverse curl has only a limited impact on the abdominal muscles because it works mainly the iliopsoas. Also, a common error when people do the traditional reverse curl is the tendency to use jerky, rocking movements to bring the knees towards the chest. Such a movement pulls the spine, because it fails to allow the iliopsoas muscle to work synergistically.

Although the rectus abdominus is the prime mover in the reverse squeeze, the transverse abdominus muscle is being worked simultaneously because of the way I have sequenced the exercise. When working on the transverse squeeze, the transverse abdominus muscle is engaged before progressing to the reverse squeeze. Since the transverse abdominus inserts into the pubis via the rectus abdominus, engaging the rectus abdominus at the second stage and maintaining the breathing rhythm and technique keeps the transverse abdominus engaged.

Reverse Abdominal Squeeze, Legs Straight

Once the reverse-squeeze technique is comfortably mastered, you can progress further by straightening both legs, keeping the knees soft or slightly bent. You could sequence this exercise as a third stage in your abdominal routine, moving on to it without a break, or you could take a breather before getting into the correct position (this time with the legs straight). This is a more intense workout for the lower abdominal area because of the greater resistance provided by the straight legs.

- Keeping the legs extended towards the ceiling, contract the lower abdominal muscles by breathing out and letting the navel sink toward the back of the spine. This time the contraction of the lower abdominal muscles will result in a slight upward push of both feet; the pubic bone will also tilt upward.

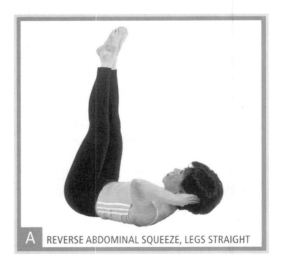

A REVERSE ABDOMINAL SQUEEZE, LEGS STRAIGHT

- Pause and then release. Vary the time that the contraction is held, and repeat for as many cycles as can be sustained.

Moon Walk I

 • Progress even further by moving alternating legs in a walking motion, with feet extended toward the ceiling.

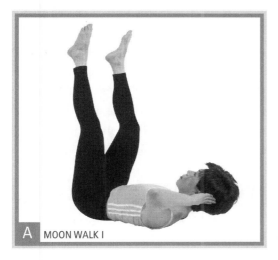

A | MOON WALK I

• With each step, breathe out to contract the abdominal muscles, letting the navel sink toward the back of the spine, and then breathe in to release before switching to the other foot. The stronger you are, the bigger the steps you can take; nevertheless, all the movements should remain slow and controlled.

• Do not swing your legs. Concentrate and focus on the abdominal muscles. The hip and back position should be absolutely stable; this is achieved by maintaining the breathing rhythm. Big steps increase the likelihood of the small of the back coming off the floor, because they affect the ability of the iliopsoas muscle to hold the hips in a stable position. Should this happen, come off the position immediately, bring both knees to the chest, hold, and rest. Once comfortable, start again. There should be no stress on the back at all.

• Repeat as many times as can be sustained.

Moon Walk II

• The next progression is to push each shoulder alternately toward the opposite leg as it is in motion, supporting the head with the hands and keeping the elbows wide and open. This exercise also works the obliques. Take care not to pull an elbow toward the oppo-

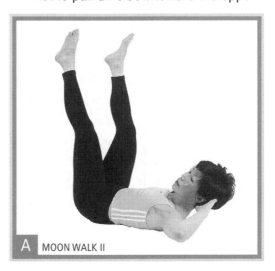

A | MOON WALK II

site leg. A violent and jerky move could injure the back or neck.

This series of movements works all four abdominal-muscle groups. As mentioned earlier, you can do them separately, as in a beginner's class, with a rest between exercises and continued checks on the body's position, or you can run through all or a selection of them in a continuous sequence. Much will depend upon the fitness of the participants.

The Pelvic Floor

One final element can be added to the lower-torso workout: pelvic-floor exercises. Fitness of the pelvic floor is vital in order to avoid problems of incontinence. This is especially true for women, who often endure tearing of these muscles during childbirth.

Pelvic-Floor Exercise

- Lie face-up with knees bent and feet firmly on the floor.

- Breathe out to contract deeply and low in the pelvic area. As you contract, the pubic bone tilts up slightly. Imagine that you are trying to stop a flow of urine; do so by squeezing all the muscles around the pelvic floor upward.

- Then release, breathing in.

This movement can be incorporated into the transverse abdominal squeeze, de-scribed on pages 105–106. To do so, combine the squeezing together of the knees with the pelvic-floor contraction.

The Obliques: Working the Waist

To eliminate excess weight around the waist, I suggest additional exercises for the obliques. A conditioned rectus abdominus and transverse abdominus helps, but the internal and external obliques should also be toned. The exercises for the obliques, based on conventional methods, have been modified to ensure that the spine is kept stable.

Side Reaches

- Lie on your back with knees bent, feet hip distance apart and slightly away from your bottom.

- Take a deep breath and exhale, letting your navel sink toward your spine and resting the small of your back on the floor.

- Breathe in again. This time, as you breathe out, raise the trunk and shoulders off the floor.

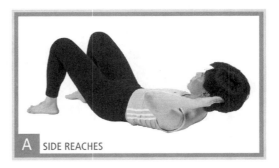

A   SIDE REACHES

▪ Breathing normally, support the head with one hand, keeping your face toward the ceiling. Reach down along one side with the other hand, as though you were trying to touch the side of your foot. It is important to keep both shoulders equidistant from the floor so they are not lop-

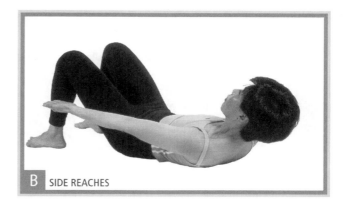

B SIDE REACHES

sided. Breathe out as you reach down, and breathe in as you return to neutral.

▪ Repeat until you feel the overload, and then change sides.

Shoulder to Knee

▪ Lie in the same position. Take a deep breath and exhale, letting your navel sink toward the back of the spine and resting the small of your back on the floor.

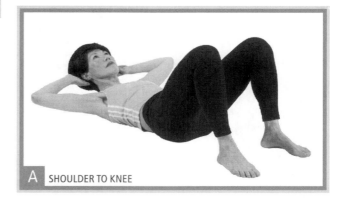

A SHOULDER TO KNEE

▪ On the next out breath raise the shoulders, supporting the head with both hands and keeping the elbows pointing outward. This is your starting position.

▪ In a controlled, smooth movement, push one shoulder toward the opposite knee, letting the other shoulder rest on the floor to give the upper trunk

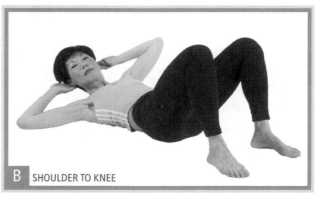

B SHOULDER TO KNEE

support and stability. Breathe out as you push toward the opposite knee, and breathe in as you return to neutral. Keep your body fully square, facing the ceiling. Be careful not to round the back or pull the elbows forward.

With this exercise I prefer to work one side at a time. Moving from side to side is less safe because the changes can become jerky, increasing the chance of damage to the back muscles. If you wish to work alternating sides, always come back to the center between contractions. For example, from the starting position, come up to the center, then contract to the left, move back to center, and then contract to the right. This way, the angle of the swing is smaller, allowing improved control.

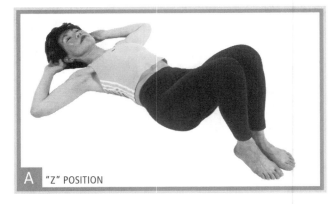

A   "Z" POSITION

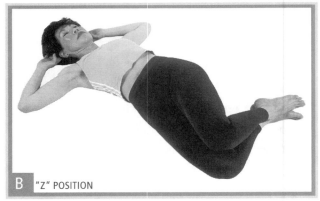

B   "Z" POSITION

"Z" Position

 ▪ Lie on your back with knees together and feet on the ground, but slightly further away from the bottom than in the side reach.

 ▪ Take a deep breath, exhale, and lower both knees to one side, preferably coming to rest on the floor. If the position is difficult or uncomfortable, or if you have back problems, rest

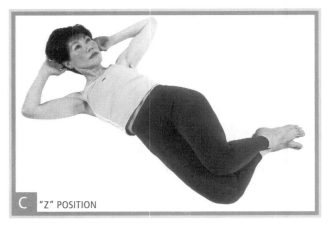

C   "Z" POSITION

your knees on a rolled towel to avoid putting pressure on the back. Placing the feet further away from the bottom than in the other two oblique exercises also helps reduce the angle of the drop when you bring the knees down. Try to keep the knees together and the upper trunk squarely facing the ceiling. Do not pull to one side.

 ■ Place your hands on each side of the head, with elbows out wide, and raise and lower your trunk, breathing out as you come up and in as you go down. Both the external and internal obliques will be engaged. Keeping the top knee down also works the adductors (inner thigh muscle) of the top leg. Repeat until you feel the overload.

■ Change sides and repeat the same sequence.

■ Introduce variations, such as coming up for two counts and down for two counts, or up for one and down for three (lengthening the time of the eccentric phase). Vary the speed of the workout.

■ You can increase the overload by raising the trunk and then reaching upward with alternating hands as though pulling on a rope. This increases the intensity on the obliques and also works the latissimus dorsi. Avoid letting the tummy bulge outward in any of these movements; do this by maintaining proper position, with the small of the back on the floor and the abdominal muscles contracted.

The Back Muscles: Erector Spinae

The *erector spinae* is a complex muscle that arises from the sacroiliac crest, the lower thoracic spine, and the spinous process. It forms a strong muscle mass that continues upward to divide into three columns of muscle, inserting into the upper ribs, the spinous process, and the cervical spine. The muscle contracts to bend the body backward or sideward and also helps rotate the spine. The erector spinae is the opposing muscle group to the abdominal muscles. It is as-

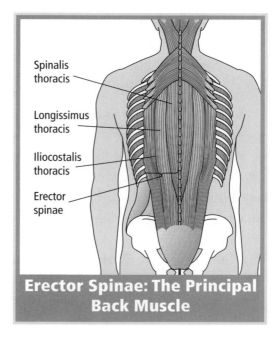

Spinalis thoracis

Longissimus thoracis

Iliocostalis thoracis

Erector spinae

Erector Spinae: The Principal Back Muscle

sisted by the transversospinalis-multifidus (see page 93). The multifidus is a series of paired small muscles extending the full length of the spine, each spanning two or three vertebrae. It is responsible for the lateral flexion, rotation, extension, and hyperextension of the spine. It also helps to stabilize the spine by keeping the vertebrae aligned.

Back Extension

- To strengthen the erector spinae, lie face down on the floor with both arms stretched out in front, or place your hands by the side of your head in the same manner as for the abdominal exercises. Your legs are extended behind you, resting on the floor.

- Take a deep breath and then exhale, keeping the hips firmly on the floor and weight evenly distributed.

- Keeping both legs still, lift the trunk off the floor in a slow, controlled motion, breathing out as you rise and breathing in as you descend.

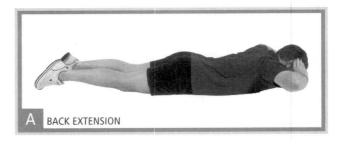

A BACK EXTENSION

- Repeat as many times as is comfortable.

Gently tilting the pelvis forward at the start of this exercise prevents the pinching of the small of the back and keeps the hip joint stable. The head comes slightly off the floor when the trunk is lifted, but avoid overextending the neck. The face should be facing the floor. It is best to pause between sets of repeats in order to avoid fatigue and poor form. This is true for all of the muscle exercises, but particularly for this one; the position is not a comfortable one because the movements exert pressure on the abdomen.

The Buttocks and Outer Thigh Muscles: Abductors

The muscles that make up the buttocks consist of the *gluteus maximus*, *gluteus medius*, and *gluteus minimus*. The gluteus maximus is responsible

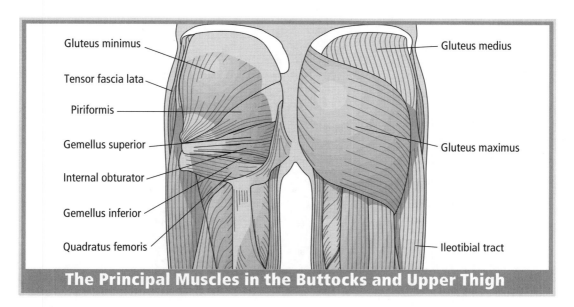

Gluteus minimus

Tensor fascia lata

Piriformis

Gemellus superior

Internal obturator

Gemellus inferior

Quadratus femoris

Gluteus medius

Gluteus maximus

Ileotibial tract

The Principal Muscles in the Buttocks and Upper Thigh

for the extension of the leg backward (back leg lifts). The gluteus medius and minimus, together with the outer thigh muscle, the *tensor fascia lata*, are responsible for carrying the leg backward and outward. Beneath the gluteals are the muscles responsible for lateral rotation of the hip. Of these, the *quadratus femoris* lies at the lowest end of the buttocks.

Firming the Buttocks: Gluteus Maximus

The conventional way of conditioning the bottom is to focus on the gluteus maximus, the biggest and most powerful muscle in the buttocks. I have adapted a widely used method of working this muscle by incorporating features of body alignment that maximize its effectiveness and make it safer.

Back Leg Lift

- Kneel, making sure that the hips are ali gned above the knees. Breathing normally, rest your elbows on the floor and align them directly below the shoulder. Make sure that the weight of the body is evenly distributed and that you are not leaning heavily to one side or the other. Your face should be looking downward; the head should be neither hanging down limp nor raised so that the neck is hyperextended. Your spine is now in a "normal" alignment.

- Exhale to tuck in the tummy, round the back slightly toward the ceiling, and tilt the pelvis slightly forward to give extra body resistance to the workout and to ensure that the small of the back does not sag.

- C ▪ Extend one leg behind you; now lift the extended leg just off the floor. This is your start position.

- D ▪ In a slow and controlled movement, lift the leg higher, pause, and then lower to starting position. The lift should be sufficient to tighten the buttocks muscles, but not so high as to cause sagging or pinching of the small of the back. Breathe out as you lift the leg, and breathe in as you lower it.

  ▪ Repeat as many times as is comfortable. Vary the speed of the contraction.

The upward motion of the leg reflects the concentric contraction of the gluteus maximus because the gluteus has its point of origin in the ilium and sacrum and inserts into the femur. The downward motion is the eccentric contraction of the muscle.

You will note that as you extend the leg behind you and lift the foot off the floor, the back returns to its normal position. If the back is not rounded and the pelvis not tilted

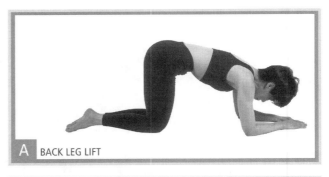

A | BACK LEG LIFT

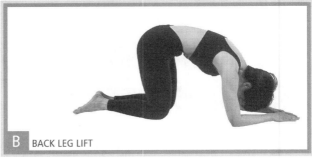

B | BACK LEG LIFT

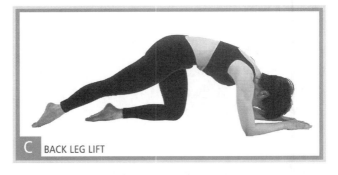

C | BACK LEG LIFT

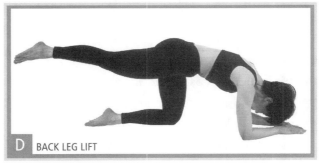

D | BACK LEG LIFT

forward at the start, the chances of the back sagging would be increased during motion. Tilting the pelvis at the beginning of movements that require the use of abductor muscles (gluteals and tensor fascia lata) help retain the normal curvature of the spine during the movement.

Side Leg Lift

 ▪ An alternative position involves lying on your side with the legs stacked on top of each other and the body aligned. Exhale, sending the navel toward the back of the spine, and gently tilt the hips forward to increase resistance and stabilize the hip joint. Some people find it easier to bend the bottom leg to obtain greater stability; for this option, make sure the knees remain in alignment with each other and with the hip.

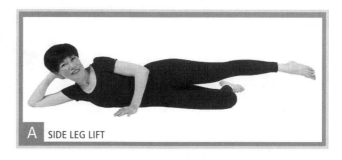

A   SIDE LEG LIFT

 ▪ Lift and lower the top leg in a slow and controlled movement. Breathe out as you lift and in as you lower. Again, the upward motion is the concentric contraction of the gluteals and the downward motion is the eccentric contraction. The tensor fascia lata is also involved; it contracts to bring the leg away from the body in the uplift.

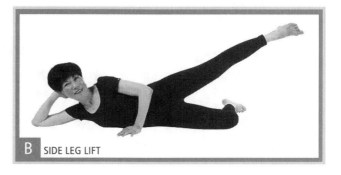

B   SIDE LEG LIFT

Erasing the Sag: Sequential Contractions

Strengthening the gluteals will help improve muscle tone in the buttocks. This is not disputed. However, except in individuals who lead a very sedentary life, the gluteals are among the most active muscles in the body because they are actively engaged in activities that involve moving the legs. Why, then, do people who are not overweight and who are reasonably active get bottoms that sag or bulge outward where the thigh joins the hip? The explanation lies at least partly in the condition of the relatively neglected lateral hip-rotating muscles, such as the quadratus femoris, which extend around the bottom of the buttock and the tensor fascia lata (see muscle diagram on page 115). The following exercises focus on the muscles of this region, especially the quadratus femoris, to help tone and support the bottom. (Other muscles in this region include the *gemellus inferior*, situated above the quadratus femoris.) These are some of the most effective methods for toning the bottom and losing the sag, and it is well worth getting the techniques right.

Straight-back Leg Extension

 ■ Lie on your right side with the left leg stacked on top of the right and the body aligned. The legs should be straight but relaxed.

 ■ Turn the body, without changing its alignment, to face the floor. Rest both forearms on the floor in front of you with the hands close together, palms down, and the elbows pointed out. You should be comfortable in this position.

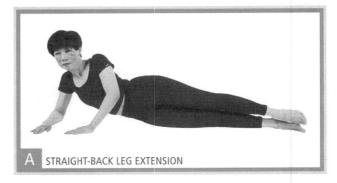

A STRAIGHT-BACK LEG EXTENSION

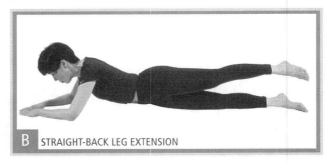

B STRAIGHT-BACK LEG EXTENSION

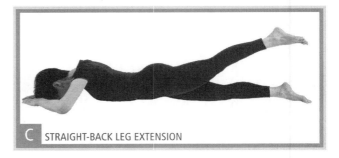

C STRAIGHT-BACK LEG EXTENSION

- Rest the face and torso on the floor, but keep the left hip just off the floor. The left knee faces down and the left leg is straight but relaxed. The right side of the body is resting comfortably on the floor.

- Inhale, and then exhale to let the navel sink toward the spine and hold in the tummy. Now tilt the hip gently forward to add body resistance to the workout; this will also help stabilize the pelvic joint and prevent the small of the back from sagging.

 - Lift and lower the left leg in a slow and controlled movement, breathing out as you lift and in as you lower. The movement should be kept fairly small.

- Vary the speed of the contractions as you progress. Instead of up for one count and down for one, go up for two and down for two, etc. This movement works the gluteals, mainly the gluteus maximus.

Right-angle Lift

- Now pause while the leg is lifted and, keeping the leg in position, turn on your side so that the left hip is stacked on top of the right hip and facing front. You may wish to come up onto your elbow and support your head by resting it on the right hand.

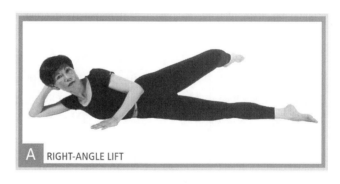

A RIGHT-ANGLE LIFT

- Bend the top leg at a 90-degree angle, keeping the calf parallel to the floor

- Lift and lower the top leg in a slow and controlled movement, again breathing out as you lift and in as you lower. You should immediately feel an impact on the outer part of the leg where it meets the line of the bottom. Again, vary the speed of the contractions as you progress. This works the tensor fascia lata and the three gluteals.

Acute Angle Moving In

- At the end of the lift, pause and turn the knee out, towards the ceiling, with the toes pointing down—a lateral rotation of the femur to engage the quadratus femoris.

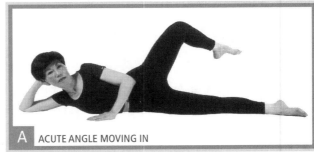

A   ACUTE ANGLE MOVING IN

- Maintain the body alignment—tummy tight, hips stable—and move the leg down toward the floor a few inches behind the supporting leg. Tilt the hip gently forward to keep the hip joint stable and to prevent the workout from turning into a hip-flexor movement.

To exercise the other buttock, start the above series lying on your left side.

In all three exercises, the body should be balanced and the movements controlled. You should not feel any discomfort. The workout is focused just beneath the bottom, toward the outer part of the thigh. The gluteals, tensor fascia lata, and quadratus femoris are all involved. You should feel the impact, even 24 hours later!

Other techniques exist to firm the buttocks, among them the buttock lift. An ancestor of the exercise that follows was popular in the 1960s and 1970s, but it fell out of favor, like many of the exercises used in that period, because it was considered too extreme. The adverse effects were considered to exceed the benefits. The most serious complaint was the stress exerted by the exercise on the small of the back. The modified version that follows has been adjusted to eliminate this and other problems presented by the traditional buttock lift.

Modified Buttock Lift

- Lie on your back with your knees bent and feet hip distance apart and placed slightly away from the bottom. The upper trunk should feel comfortable and relaxed.

- Breathe in, and then exhale, bringing the navel toward the spine. This allows the abdomen to flatten and the pelvis to stabilize.

- On the next out-breath, lift the buttocks slightly higher than fist height off the floor. This is the starting position. Be careful not to lift the buttocks too high by arching the small of the back.

- Squeeze the buttocks upward, and then release by gently lowering them to their starting position. Breathe out as you lift and in as you lower. The movements are slow and controlled, the back should not arch up, and there should be no stress on the back.

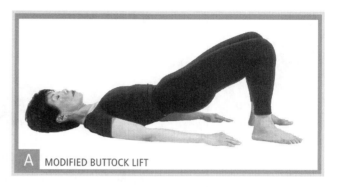

A MODIFIED BUTTOCK LIFT

- Repeat until you feel the overload.

Modifications can be made to this position so that you are working the tensor fascia latae (outer thigh) and the adductors (inner thigh).

- At the end of the up-lift, pause to check that the back is correctly aligned (i.e., not pinching), and then squeeze the knees in to touch each other, breathing out as you do so. The feet remain hip-distance apart.

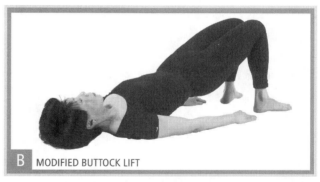

B MODIFIED BUTTOCK LIFT

- Release, breathing in, and move the knees apart.

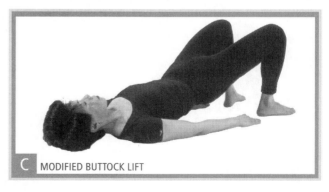

C MODIFIED BUTTOCK LIFT

- Repeat as many times as you can sustain. You will notice a tightening of the inner thigh muscles and the upper end of the outer thigh just below the bottom.

You can progress even further as follows:

D - Walk your feet inward until they are together.

- With knees closed, squeeze the buttocks upward, pause, and release them down. Again, breathe out as you squeeze up and in as you release.

- Repeat.

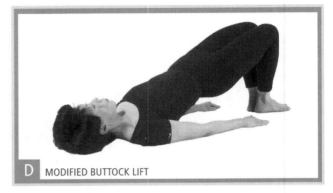

D MODIFIED BUTTOCK LIFT

The intensity of the workout on the gluteals, tensor fascia latae, and adductors is noticeable to say the least. I have grown to enjoy the sensation and particularly its effect!

The Inner Thigh Muscles: Adductors

Adductors, located in the inner thigh, are responsible for moving the leg inward, hip flexion, and lateral rotation of the hip. They consist of four muscles: the *pectineus*, *adductor brevis*, *adductor longus*, and *adductor magnus*. They originate from the pubic bone and the lower part of the hip bone and insert into the femur.

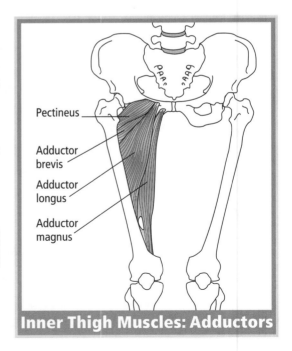

Pectineus

Adductor brevis

Adductor longus

Adductor magnus

Inner Thigh Muscles: Adductors

Inner Thigh Seesaw: Toning the Inner Thigh

- Lie on your side with legs extended, one on top of the other, making sure that the body is completely aligned.

The upper trunk can rest on the floor, or it may be more comfortable to support the head.

 ▪ Keeping the lower leg extended, bend the top leg and bring it over until the knee rests on the floor. Those with back problems might need to rest the knee on a rolled towel. The extended leg should be straight, with the knee soft.

 ▪ Lift and lower the extended leg. Lift as high as can be comfortably sustained. The movement should be slow and controlled. The intensity can be increased by reducing the speed of the movements, especially when lowering the leg. Pausing at the end of the lift also increases the intensity. Again, breathe out as you lift and in as you lower. Don't touch the floor with your foot when you come down—and keep the stomach muscles in good control!

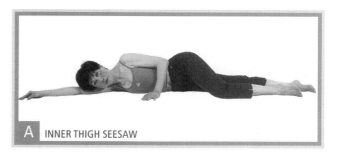

A INNER THIGH SEESAW

I have increased the intensity of this exercise in more advanced classes by adding the following variation, which involves the use of the obliques:

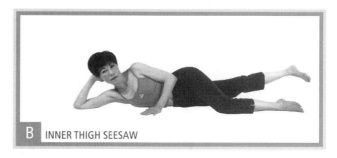

B INNER THIGH SEESAW

 ▪ As the lower leg is lifted, reach towards the lifted foot with the upper arm, effecting an oblique crunch. Breathe out as you reach toward the lifted leg.

▪ When the leg goes down, release the crunch, breathing in as you do so. Allow the arm to return to its starting position.

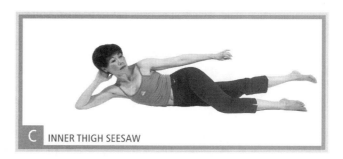

C INNER THIGH SEESAW

- Repeat as many times as can be sustained. Add variation by changing the speed of the movements, for example, going up for two and down for two, up for one and down for three, and vice versa.

The Quadriceps

This group of muscles is situated in the front thigh. It consists of the *rectus femoris*, the largest and most powerful in the group; *vastus lateralis*; *vastus medialis*; and *vastus intermedius*. The rectus femoris originates from the front point of the ilium, and the others originate in the upper portion of the femur. All four muscles insert into the tibia via the patellar ligament. The rectus femoris contracts, flexing the thigh at the hip to lift the leg. The iliopsoas (hip flexor muscle) is also involved in the process. All of the quadriceps muscles work the knee joint and are responsible for movements involving knee extension, such as straightening the lower leg.

The most common way to exercise the quadriceps is through squats. Note, however, that in all of the exercises for the quadriceps that follow, the iliopsoas is also involved.

Conventional Squats

- Stand with your legs hip distance apart, feet facing front.

- Keeping the stomach muscles tight and back straight, bend your knees

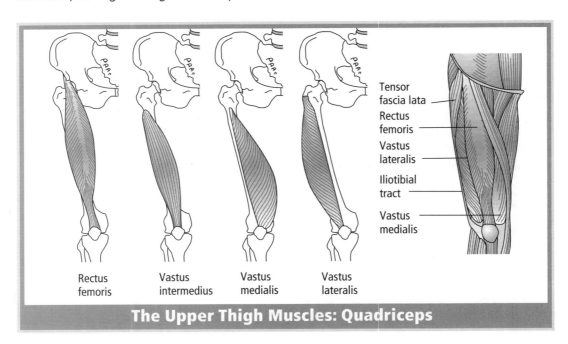

Rectus femoris   Vastus intermedius   Vastus medialis   Vastus lateralis

Tensor fascia lata
Rectus femoris
Vastus lateralis
Iliotibial tract
Vastus medialis

The Upper Thigh Muscles: Quadriceps

until your bottom is above the knees at an angle of about 45 degrees (be sure to avoid dropping the bottom lower than the knees).

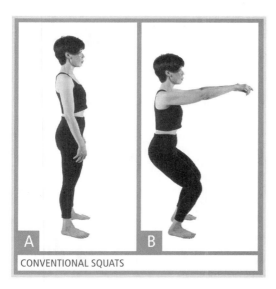

CONVENTIONAL SQUATS

- Straighten your legs slowly to return to an upright position. Breathe out as you lower and in as you straighten up. I find that greater resistance is obtained if, when straightening the legs, you tilt the pelvis slightly forward (keeping the tummy tucked in), as though you were squeezing up. This helps to stabilize the hips as well.

- Repeat until you feel the overload.

A number of variations on the squat exist, including:

- Ski squats, in which the bottom is pushed back and the trunk is inclined forward.

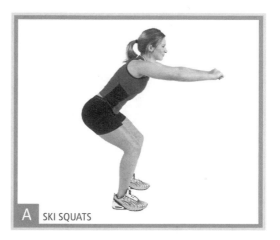

A SKI SQUATS

- Travel squats, in which you squat to one side and then drag the leg back to the center (this also exercises the adductors).

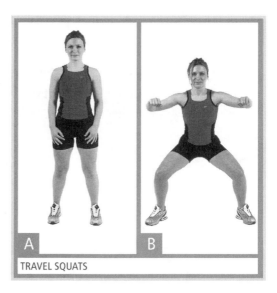

TRAVEL SQUATS

Pedal and Stride

Pedal-and-stride exercises offer an alternative way of strengthening the quadriceps.

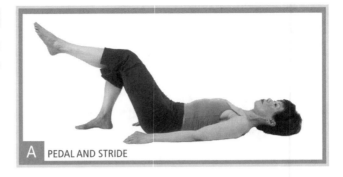

A PEDAL AND STRIDE

- Lie on your back on the floor, with knees bent and both feet on the floor.

- Breathe in, and then exhale to let the navel sink toward the back of the spine.

Ⓐ Keeping the tummy muscles controlled, on the next out-breath raise one leg off the ground. The knee of the raised leg should be slightly bent. This is your starting position.

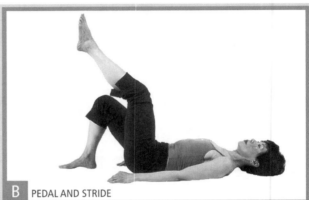

B PEDAL AND STRIDE

Ⓑ In a slow and controlled man-ner, lift the leg higher, pause, and then lower the leg, taking care that your foot does not touch the floor. Breathe out as you lift and in as you lower.

- Repeat as many times as is comfortable. The working leg remains slightly bent, keeping the angle of the bend unchanged when lifting and lowering. A further variation of this exercise would be to bend and straighten the leg.

If you are a more advanced student, you might wish to skip the pre-ceding and start with the following:

- Lift your upper trunk, supporting it with your elbows resting on the floor and aligned below the shoulders. Shoulders are relaxed. The knees are bent and both feet are on the floor. Make sure that you face front and that your head is not tilted back.

- Breathe in, and then exhale to let your navel sink toward the spine. Retain control of the stomach muscles.

- On the next out-breath, raise one leg off the floor, with the knee slightly bent. This is your starting position.

- Raise and lower the leg, without changing the angle of the bent knee, in a slow and controlled manner. Breathe out as you lift and in as you lower. Add variation by changing the speed and counts going up and down. Further variation would be to bring the knee in towards the chest and then to fully extend the leg, leading with the heel.

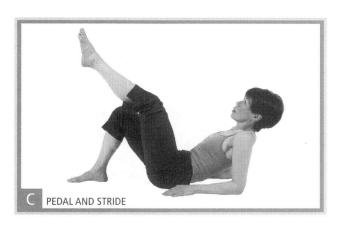

C PEDAL AND STRIDE

- Repeat until you feel the overload on the quadriceps.

By now, you should feel a significant load on the muscle and you might need a break. If you are very strong and wish to progress even more, go to the next step, which is a very advanced position and

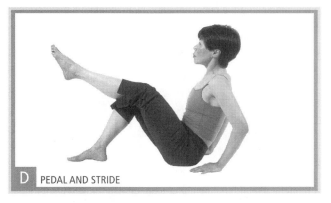

D PEDAL AND STRIDE

should be attempted only if your abdominal muscles are very strong.

- Bring the trunk up even further to almost a sitting position, and carry out the same moves to stabilize the hip and engage the transverse abdominal muscles. Breathe in, and then exhale to let the navel sink toward the spine. Make sure your lower back remains stabilized, neither arching upward nor rounding back toward the floor; additionally, don't let your tummy bulge outward. Do this by keeping your abdominal muscles properly engaged.

D ▪ Lift and lower the leg, as before, with as many repeats as you can sustain.

This position develops resistance as the angle between the leg and the trunk becomes more acute, increasing the leverage and making it harder to lift the leg. To do this exercise without stressing the back requires great strength and control in the abdominal muscles because they must hold the trunk in position, in order not to stress the spine. Position D is not recommended for beginners or intermediate students, or for those who have not mastered the abdominal exercises described above.

The Barre

This exercise is invaluable because it contributes to a strong and toned upper leg or quadriceps, which both looks good and

helps avoid knee problems. Borrowed from ballet practices, it requires the use of the barre—or some other support that is stable, strong, and above waist height, such as a wall. It involves very controlled and strong movements and is not for the feint-hearted! You can, however, work at your level and build up strength to move to the most advanced stage.

▪ Stand sideways slightly away from the barre or wall, and rest the nearest hand on it for support. A

▪ Bring the knee of the outer leg up towards the chest, supporting it with the free hand clasped around the back of the thigh. Check that you are completely stable. B

▪ Bend the body toward the lifted leg, keeping the knee of the standing leg

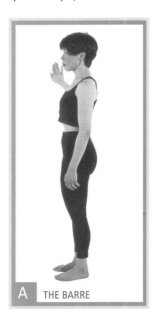

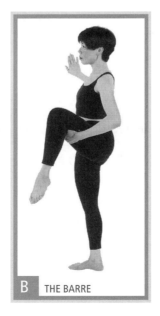

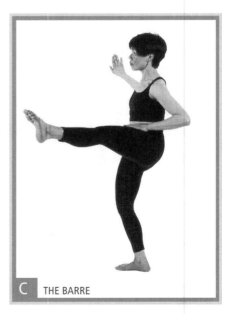

A THE BARRE

B THE BARRE

C THE BARRE

soft. This increases the intensity of the exercise but reduces the stress on the supporting leg. This is your starting position.

- Pointing the toes, extend the raised leg sideways at an angle of about 45 degrees, raising it as high as is comfortable. Now straighten the raised leg. It's very tempting once you straighten the leg to allow the hips to release, the pelvis to roll back, and the knee of the extended leg to rotate toward the front. Instead, keep the hips tucked under and the knee facing upward. If necessary, bring the leg a little lower to maintain good form, which is essential if you want to work the targeted muscles.

- Pause, then bend the leg to release. Keep all movements slow and controlled.

- Repeat as many times as can be sustained.

To start with, it is preferable to keep the number of reps in each set small, so that you can have a breather between sets. Vary the angle and size of the bends to get a change in resistance. You can execute the same moves with the leg extended in front rather than to the side, which will change the emphasis of the workload to different quadriceps muscles.

This exercise is deceptively hard. When I first did it, I realized that I was not as strong as I thought. The ache that followed was incredible, as I had done the sets at a height that was obviously beyond me at that time. It is important not to have the leg so high that you cannot sustain the movement or you feel excessive strain. The higher the leg, the greater the resistance applied to the quadriceps, and the more difficult the exercise. Work towards greater height, but do not start with it. Pointing the toes when you extend the leg will also work the arch of the foot, which is often neglected. This is a wonderful upper-leg shaper and well worth the effort.

The Hamstring

This group of muscles, consisting of the *semitendinosus*, *semimembranosus*, and

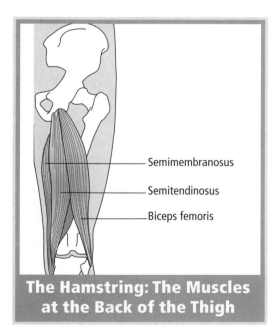

The Hamstring: The Muscles at the Back of the Thigh

Semimembranosus

Semitendinosus

Biceps femoris

biceps femoris, is located at the back of the leg. The point of origin is the ischial tuberosity (bottom of the pelvis, the ischium) and the back of the femur, and it inserts into the tibia. The hamstring contracts to flex the knee, bringing the heel towards the bottom and lengthening the muscles at the front of the thigh.

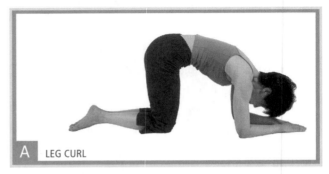

A · LEG CURL

Leg Curl

One of the most common floor exercises for this muscle group is the leg curl.

 · Kneel, with your elbows resting on the floor. Make sure that the hips are aligned above the knee and the elbows are aligned below the shoulders. Keep your weight evenly distributed.

· On the next out-breath, pull the tummy in to help straighten the back and keep it from sagging. This position also enhances the body resistance when working the hamstring.

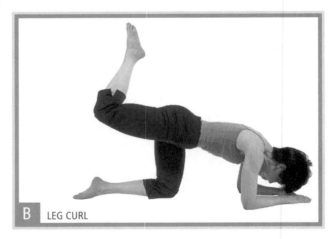

B · LEG CURL

B · Breathe in, and as you exhale, bring one knee off the floor, so that the foot faces the ceiling.

C · Breathe normally to straighten and bend the leg in a slow and controlled way. It is important not to push the knee/leg too high, because this will cause

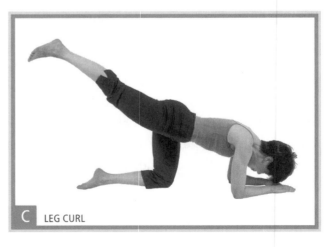

C · LEG CURL

the small of the back to sag and exert excessive pressure on the hip joint.

- Repeat to achieve the overload, and then change sides.

Variations include straightening in two phases and bending in two phases.

The Calf and Shin Muscles: Gastrocnemius, Soleus, and Tibialis Anterior

The *gastrocnemius* is the powerful calf muscle, which originates at the back of the femur, just above the knee, and inserts via a tendon into the Achilles calcaneous. It is supported by the *soleus*, which originates in the tibia, just below the knee, and also inserts via a tendon into the Achilles calcaneus. Both muscles contract to flex the heel, causing the toes to point, referred to as *plantar flexion*. The opposing muscle group is the *tibialis anterior*, located in front of the leg. Originating from the front of the tibia, just below the knee, it inserts into the inner edge of the foot. Contraction causes the foot to flex upwards, referred to as *dorsi flexion*.

Working these muscles involves moves that result in plantar and dorsi flexion. For example, raising and lowering the heel works the calf muscles. Flexing the foot works the tibialis anterior. The calves are worked intensively in daily activities such as walking, running, and going up or down stairs. Most aerobic routines involve them.

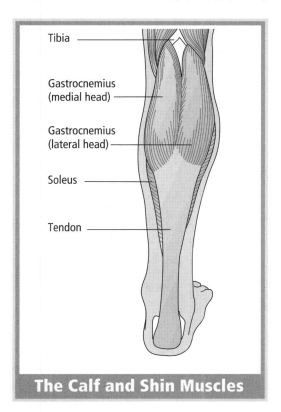

Tibia

Gastrocnemius (medial head)

Gastrocnemius (lateral head)

Soleus

Tendon

The Calf and Shin Muscles

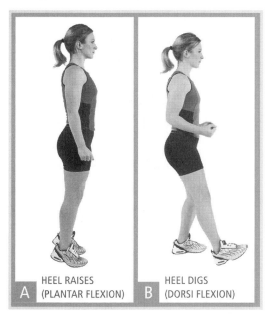

A HEEL RAISES (PLANTAR FLEXION)

B HEEL DIGS (DORSI FLEXION)

In step classes, they are the most worked of all the muscles. Therefore, I have included only these two moves for them.

Upper Torso and Arms

The Chest Muscles: Pectoralis Major and Minor

Pectoralis is the Latin word for "breast." There are two groups of pectoral muscles: the *pectoralis major* and the *pectoralis minor*. The pectoralis major is a large fan-shaped muscle that covers most of the chest and is responsible for the movement of the arms inward and

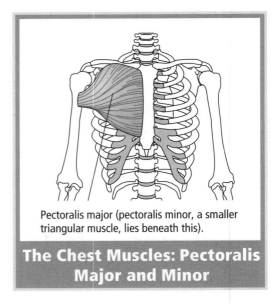

Pectoralis major (pectoralis minor, a smaller triangular muscle, lies beneath this).

The Chest Muscles: Pectoralis Major and Minor

across the body. It originates from the clavicle and sternum and the adjacent parts of the second to the sixth ribs and inserts into the humerus. The pectoralis minor is a smaller muscle beneath the pectoralis major. It originates from the third to the fifth ribs and inserts into the scapula (shoulder blade), which it moves down and forward.

The pectoral muscles are a major source of muscular strength and feature widely in strength and endurance training, especially for men. They are important for women because they provide vital support for the breasts. The most common method for training this muscle for endurance and strength is the floor push-up. I provide three versions here, devised according to different levels of strength.

Push-ups

- Kneel and place both hands on the floor with the knees aligned below the hips. The hands are kept fairly wide apart to maximize the impact on the pectoralis and for balance.

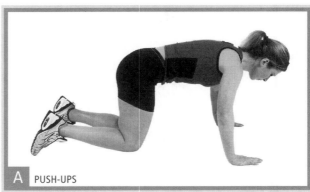

A PUSH-UPS

B ▪ Hold the tummy in so that the back does not sag, then bend your arms to lower the chest to just above the floor.

▪ Raise the torso by straightening the arms. Breathe in while you're pressing up and breathe out, tucking the tummy in, while you're lowering down. (Breathing out while lowering the body helps prevent the small of the back from sagging.) It should be noted, however, that some schools of thought recommend breathing out while pressing up.

C ▪ To increase the intensity of the workout, extend the legs further behind so that more weight and resistance is shifted to the chest, and execute the same moves.

D ▪ To increase the body resistance even more, extend both legs fully.

Progression is achieved by varying the speed of the contraction. The muscle meets greater resistance if the chest is lowered slowly, with a pause at each phase of descent.

Many variations of the push-up exist, but they are not usually recommended for the average person because they are potentially dangerous.

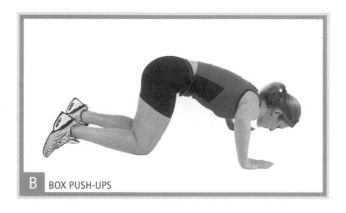

B | BOX PUSH-UPS

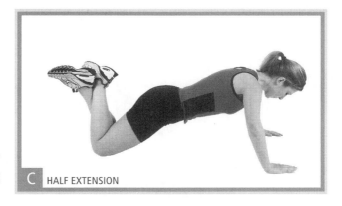

C | HALF EXTENSION

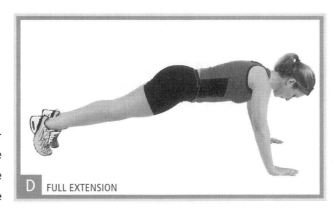

D | FULL EXTENSION

They include combining floor push-ups with ballistic moves such as taking both hands off the floor to clap between push-ups, or the inverted push-up, where the hands are turned inward with the fingers touching. Floor push-ups also strengthen the triceps, biceps, and deltoids.

The Chest Press

The chest press provides a convenient way of exercising the pectoral muscles:

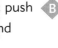

- Grasp the opposite wrist with each hand and push inward to the medial line of the chest; or, alternatively, push the heel of the palms together and then release.

- Repeat until you feel the overload.

The chest press is very useful for women seeking to tone the chest muscle because it can be done practically anywhere at any time. It focuses on the area just below the shoulder joint, which is important for supporting the breasts, yet it does not put stress on the shoulder joints or require strength. The exercise is unlikely to increase strength, but done regularly it helps tone the pectoralis. To gain greater muscular strength, weight training, combined with full-floor push-ups, is generally used.

The Upper Back Muscles: Trapezius and Rhomboids

The muscles of the upper back are opposing muscles to the pectoral muscles. The *trape-zius*, a large diamond-shaped muscle in the back, stretches from the base of the skull and the shoulders down to the lower part of the thoracic spine. Its point of origin is from the seventh cervical joint to the twelfth thoracic vertebra. It inserts into the clavicle and the scapula. The trapezius helps support the neck and is responsible for the raising and adduction of the shoulders as well as the lateral flexion of the neck and its rotation. The *rhomboid*, a smaller muscle, also arises from the seventh cervical

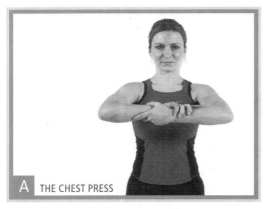

A THE CHEST PRESS

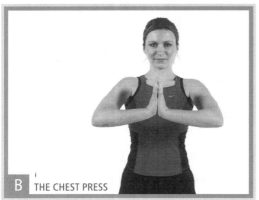

B THE CHEST PRESS

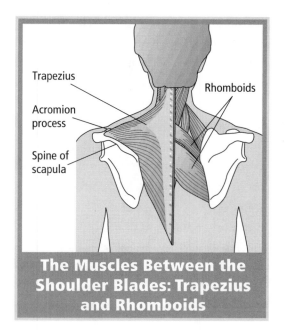

The Muscles Between the Shoulder Blades: Trapezius and Rhomboids

The trapezius and rhomboid muscles are also involved in push-ups. When the chest is lowered, the shoulder blades are pushed inward.

The Back Muscle: Latissimus Dorsi

This flat, almost triangular muscle starts from the lower spinous process (the sixth lower thoracic spine and the fifth lumbar vertebrae) and the crest of the ilium, and converges into the humerus (upper arm bone) just below the shoulders. It is primarily responsible for moving the arm downward and backward.

Exercises for the latissimus dorsi include pulling down and rowing movements. A common exercise is as follows:

vertebra and the upper five thoracic vertebrae. It inserts into the scapula and contracts to pull (adduct) toward the spine, and it also rotates the scapula. The trapezius and rhomboids tend to feel tight and strained in people who work at desk-bound jobs.

Here are some exercises for these muscles that can be done conveniently at a desk:

- Slowly circle the arms or shoulders.

- Raise both shoulders towards the ears, and then lower. Repeat several times until you feel an easing of tension in the shoulders and upper back.

- Gently squeeze the shoulder blades together.

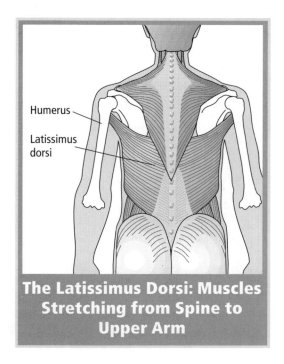

The Latissimus Dorsi: Muscles Stretching from Spine to Upper Arm

- Take hold of a bar, holding it above the head and spacing the hands well apart.

- Lower the bar, keeping it behind the head, until it is just above the shoulder. Pause, then raise the bar again to its original position.

- Repeat as many times as can be sustained in a slow and controlled manner.

This exercise also works the rhomboids and trapezius. Weights or dumbbells can be used instead of a bar.

The Arm Muscles: Deltoids, Biceps, and Triceps

These muscles are situated in the upper arm. The *deltoid* is the rounded muscle in the outer upper arm. It originates from the scapula and clavicle, and inserts into the humerus. When it contracts, it moves the arm upwards. The *biceps* is the muscle in the upper arm responsible for bending the arm towards the body, for example, when lifting an object. It also helps rotate the forearm. It originates from the scapula and inserts into the radius. Finally, the *triceps* is at the back of the upper arm. It originates from the scapula and humerus, and inserts into the ulna. It contracts to straighten the arm and is the opposing muscle group to the biceps.

In the aging process or following weight gain, the triceps tends to be the worst affected, becoming flabby and loose. The problem is more common in women, partly because few women do heavy manual

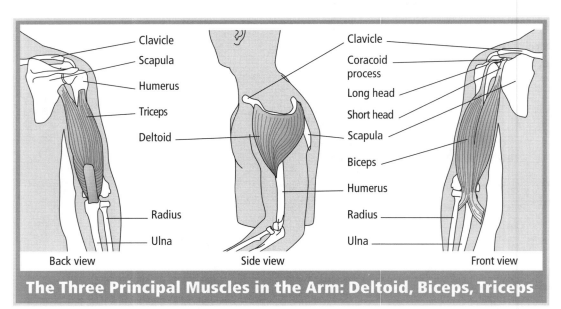

Back view · Side view · Front view

The Three Principal Muscles in the Arm: Deltoid, Biceps, Triceps

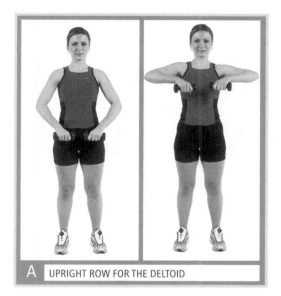

A | UPRIGHT ROW FOR THE DELTOID

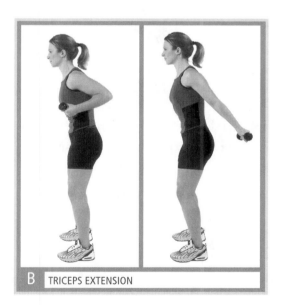

B | TRICEPS EXTENSION

Floor push-ups also involve the triceps, biceps, and deltoids. Increasing the body resistance by going into half or full push-ups increases the intensity of the workout on these muscles. Other, milder exercises for these three muscle groups using one's own

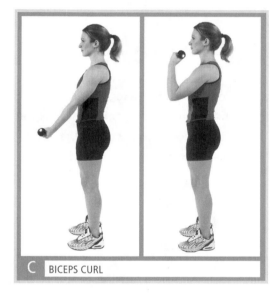

C | BICEPS CURL

body resistance include upright row for the deltoid (A), triceps extension (B), and biceps curl (C). You may wish to use weights for these exercises.

Triceps Extension on the Floor

The following is a more advanced version of the triceps extension; this variation is widely used.

work, but also for genetic reasons. In view of this, I have provided a larger range of triceps exercises than for the deltoids or the biceps.

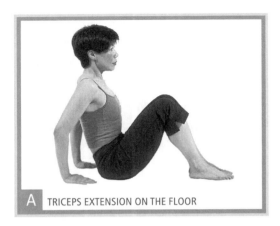

A TRICEPS EXTENSION ON THE FLOOR

A ■ Sit on the floor with legs bent and hands on the floor on either side of the body, placed slightly behind the buttocks, with the fingers facing forward.

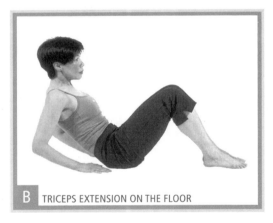

B TRICEPS EXTENSION ON THE FLOOR

■ Take a deep breath, and then exhale, letting the navel sink toward the back of the spine.

B ■ Holding the tummy in, lower the body towards the back by bending the arms, exhaling as you do so.

■ Inhale to return to a sitting position, straightening the arms.

■ To give even greater resistance from the same position, lift the buttocks off the floor, straightening the arms, and breathing in as you do so. This contracts the triceps concentrically.

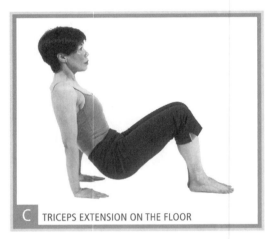

C TRICEPS EXTENSION ON THE FLOOR

■ To release, bend the arms at the elbow and lower the buttocks, breathing out. This contracts the triceps eccentrically.

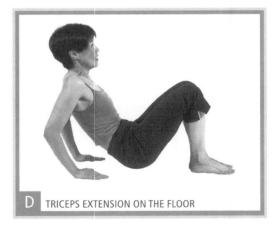

D TRICEPS EXTENSION ON THE FLOOR

Good tummy control is needed in order to protect the back and ensure that the workout is focused on the triceps. Individuals with poor stomach control or weak shoulders should not attempt to lift the buttocks off the floor (C and D), because doing so increases the force on the joints. Be careful not to jolt the shoulders.

An alternative, advanced workout for the triceps that I find very useful and that involves no weight or stress to the shoulders is as follows:

Back Arm Lifts

- Stand with your feet hip distance apart. Exhale to tuck the tummy in, and lean slightly forward.

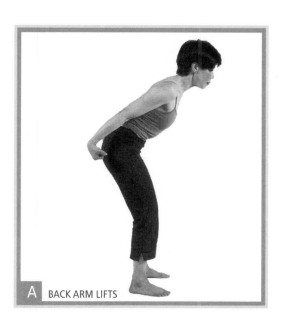

A   BACK ARM LIFTS

- Breathing normally, extend both arms straight behind you as high as is comfortable. Keep the arms and elbows tight against the body.

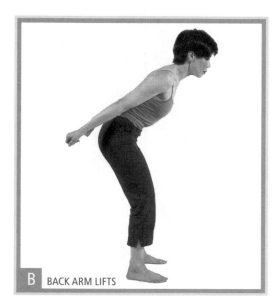

B   BACK ARM LIFTS

- With your fists lightly clenched to face downward, bend the wrists (which also bends the elbows slightly), and extend and lift your arms up and back. Breathe out as you lift and in as you release.

- Repeat until you feel the overload on the triceps.

Scissoring the Arms

- To increase the intensity of the work- out, unclench the fist at the end of the

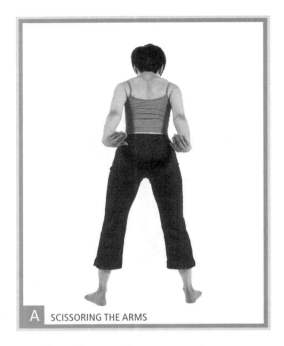

A SCISSORING THE ARMS

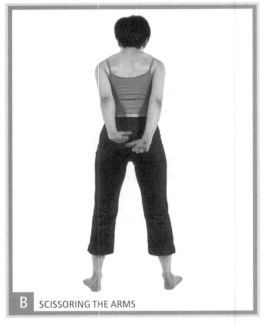

B SCISSORING THE ARMS

lift and rotate the arms so that your fingers point upwards to the ceiling.

 • Scissor the arms in big movements. Breathe normally and maintain tight tummy control throughout.

You should feel the workout on the triceps quite strongly. Regular use of this exercise will result in a marked improvement in the tone of the triceps within three weeks. For serious muscular strength and endurance training aimed at building muscle bulk, these exercises can be performed using weights.

10

Training for Flexibility: Eliminating Stress and Strain

Flexible people can bend, reach, and turn without strain or force. Their muscles are pliable and supple. Their joints are similarly mobile. However, even these fortunate individuals, who probably owe their condition to regular exercise, must confront the decline in flexibility that can come with aging. The postural muscles that support the body tend to shorten with time. This gives rise to the stooped posture of many elderly people. The muscles responsible for maintaining and generating movement can also weaken. Joints become stiff. This loss of flexibility, associated with age, can be made worse by the continuous muscle contraction associated with frequent high-intensity exercises. Sports such as running, jumping, and sprinting can contribute to the onset of tight muscles.

The tendency for flexibility to decline with age does not mean that the loss of flexibility is inevitable. It is widespread, largely because very few people stretch as part of their daily routine. Some do not even stretch at the end of a hard workout. As a result, the contracted muscles remain tight and over time become permanently so. Yet a few minutes of stretching every day will help to maintain muscle suppleness and joint mobility as well as relieve the tension and stress that can accumulate in the shoulders. You only have to watch household pets or even birds in the garden as they go through their regular stretching routines to know that this is the natural way to prepare for movement and to set the body healthily at rest after activity.

The Benefits of Stretching

Stretching improves posture, reduces back problems, and enhances the quality and grace of movements. This is easily illustrated. If you stretch up towards the ceiling after a long day spent behind a desk, you feel a wonderful lengthening of the back muscles and a release of tension. With the stretch, the vertebrae in the spinal column get a chance for space and movement, which they have been denied during the long hours of enforced sitting. This is recognized by many companies, who now include as part of their new employee orientation programs information on health and safety in which, among other things, they emphasize the need for a comfortable working position and regular breaks away from the desk to relax and stretch.

In sports, stretching helps to improve performance because it enables joints and muscles to be taken to their full range. A runner with tight shin muscles will find it hard to run uphill or sprint. Dancers cannot perform with tight hamstrings. People who play tennis, football, or similar sports that require rapid changes in direction must maintain the flexibility of the adductors. The

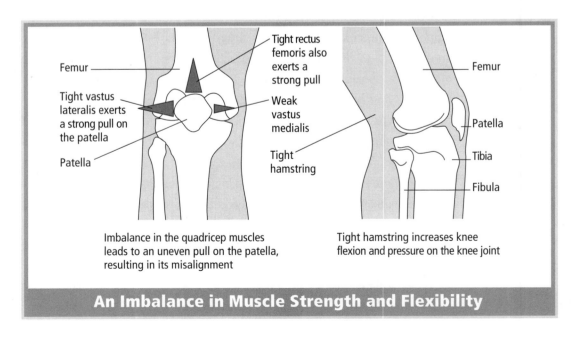

Imbalance in the quadricep muscles leads to an uneven pull on the patella, resulting in its misalignment

Tight hamstring increases knee flexion and pressure on the knee joint

An Imbalance in Muscle Strength and Flexibility

iliopsoas muscles, which are crucial for rapid changes of direction by the lower body, also need to be strong and supple.

Muscle tightness can cause serious sports injury. Stretching muscles before and after they have been worked contributes substantially to reducing injuries such as muscle tear and damage to ligaments and tendons. The impact of tight muscles is often cumulative. For the kneecap to work well, the quadriceps that hold it in position must be balanced so that it is correctly aligned. If they are not, it can be pulled out of alignment. If the hamstring is tense, it will stop the leg from being straightened. This excessive flexion of the knee, in turn, causes the kneecap to press harder on the femur. This pressure can result in inflammation and pain. The increase in the flexion of the knee caused by tight hamstrings will also lead to higher impact on the ankle as the foot lands on the ground. A tight iliotibial band (see illustration on the right), which results from overuse, can lead to pain in the lower thigh or outer knee. (For more detail, see Chapter 11, which considers sports injuries.)

Stretching each muscle after it has been involved in activity helps maintain its length and flexibility and prevents the onset of injuries. It also helps to improve coordination between opposing muscle groups. Stretching counteracts the tendency for

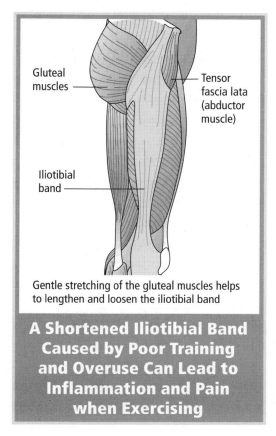

Gentle stretching of the gluteal muscles helps to lengthen and loosen the iliotibial band

A Shortened Iliotibial Band Caused by Poor Training and Overuse Can Lead to Inflammation and Pain when Exercising

muscles to bulk up following intensive training. It is especially relevant for those who do not wish to have big muscles. Finally, stretching reduces muscle soreness as the muscle returns to normal length and the buildup of lactic acid is dispersed.

Types of Stretching

In Chapter 6, I touched upon the importance of stretching prior to and following exercise. For flexibility training, these stretches have to be complemented by a fuller, more thorough stretching of muscles on the completion of the activity. The extent and nature of the stretches depends on the objective. If it is simply to return the muscle to its length before the start of the activity, then a short maintenance stretch might suffice. These could be similar to the preparatory stretches described in Chapter 6, and each should be held for around 10 to 12 seconds.

If the objective is to develop the flexibility of the muscle, then the stretches will have to be held for substantially longer. These are generally referred to as *developmental stretches*, and there is no fixed rule on how long they must be held. Instead, a rule of thumb applies: Hold the stretch until the muscle relaxes, then develop the stretch further, and hold it again for about 25 to 30 seconds, or as long as is comfortable. Avoid exerting any force. The first phase takes time, because, as explained in Chapter 3, the muscle spindles react to the initial stretch by tightening the muscles, the so-called *stretch reflex*. The faster and more abruptly a stretch is effected, the more the muscles respond by contracting rather than releasing. Hence, it is vital to go into a stretch in a slow and controlled way, paying special attention to the stability of the joints involved.

There are four groups of stretching techniques:

- ballistic stretching

- static stretching

- active stretching

- stretching against external resistance, or proprioceptive neuromuscular facilitation (PNF)

Ballistic stretching involves lengthening the muscle to the maximum that can be reached, and then bouncing to take the stretch even further. Bouncing at the end of the stretch causes the muscles to tighten in response. The greater the force of the bounce, the tighter the muscles become; the enforced strain can result in muscle tear and damage.

As a result, ballistic stretches, commonly used in the past, are now largely frowned

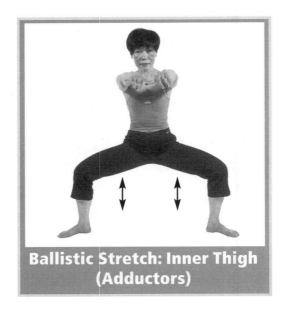

Ballistic Stretch: Inner Thigh (Adductors)

upon, except in training for competitive gymnastics. A typical ballistic stretch is as follows:

- Place the feet wide apart with knees turned out to either side.

- Lower the bottom until the muscles in the inner thigh feel stretched to their maximum.

- Bounce to lower the bottom further and increase the stretch.

In this example, the knee and hip joints are also destabilized and subjected to pressure.

Static stretching is the opposite of ballistic stretching. It is the gradual lengthening of the muscle until a stretch is felt. The stretch is held and then released; no bouncing or force is involved. This is a safe and gentle way to lengthen the muscle, using mainly gravity and the support of the body. For example, to stretch the hamstring:

- Lie on your back with the knees up, feet down on the floor.

- Bring one knee towards the chest and then straighten it upwards, supporting the leg with both hands. Keep your bottom on the floor and the extended leg straight.

The stretch is felt at the back of the thigh (hamstring) of the straightened leg, from the bottom down to the back of the

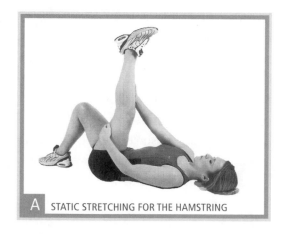

A   STATIC STRETCHING FOR THE HAMSTRING

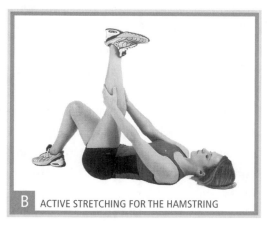

B   ACTIVE STRETCHING FOR THE HAMSTRING

knee. The muscles, both the quadriceps and the tibialis anterior, are relaxed.

Many people do not feel sufficiently stretched by static stretches. To develop the stretch further, the opposing muscle group is sometimes brought into use. Continuing with the static stretch for the hamstring, this becomes an *active stretch* if the foot of the extended leg is flexed. The back of the leg, including the hamstring and the gastrocnemius, is lengthened even more. However, because the tibialis anterior is actively engaged in flexing the foot and is shortened, the position should not be held for longer than 10 or 15 seconds. This avoids prolonged contraction and stress of the opposing muscle group. A gentle repetition of active stretches is usually preferable. Active stretches, with repetitive flex and release, are an integral part of a warm-up in most fitness classes and are considered best suited for stretching muscle groups that cross major joints, such as the hips, knees, ankles, and shoulders.

One of the safest muscle stretches uses external assistance, or PNF. This involves alternating static stretching and isometric contraction of a muscle against an object or partner. The isometric contraction should not be held for longer than six seconds. Using the example of a hamstring stretch, the extended leg of the participant lying down is supported by a partner, who holds the leg. Stretch statically against the partner, who should provide only mild assistance in the stretch (e.g., helping to gently ease the leg towards the participant), and then contract isometrically against the partner, who provides resistance against the contraction. Release after six seconds, and then repeat the stretch and contraction. Note that this approach is only safe if the partner is competent. There must be complete trust between the participants, and it

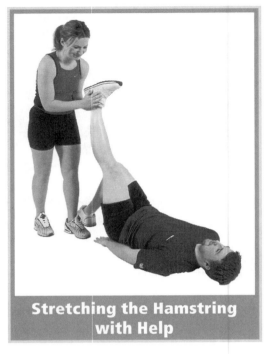

Stretching the Hamstring with Help

is preferable for many of the exercises that they be of similar height and strength.

Working with an inanimate object such as a barre can overcome some of these potential difficulties. By placing the leg on the barre and leaning forward, the hamstring can be supported as it is stretched statically without using the opposing muscle group. Make sure the barre is at the correct height. If it is too low, it exerts stress on the back; too high and it can stress the hip joint, knee, and leg.

As you can see, each of the different groups of stretching techniques has some disadvantages, but they are not insurmountable.

Training Exercises for Flexibility

Stretches require sound technique and a good understanding of one's body; otherwise they may be executed badly and cause injuries. It is important to know your body's capacity and to set sensible targets. You should stretch to your personal maximum and avoid competing with others. Unfortunately, stretching in a class tends to encourage competitiveness in part because the act of stretching is slow and gives participants time to compare and contest with each other. The reverse can also occur. Some people are so self-conscious that they avoid stretching if they possibly can. It is important to be aware of the differences that exist between people and to accept them. Then set your own objectives for flexibility training.

Objectives vary between individuals: For some it could be to maintain muscle length, for others to develop flexibility within their natural range, while a few might wish to push further. You should note that extreme stretching positions are not suitable for everyone and can be dangerous unless participants are well trained and already have a supple body. Remember that extending flexibility beyond the full natural range of movement is not necessary for normal activity. It is a personal choice.

It is extremely difficult to determine what is "natural" and what is not because of the wide differences in people's flexibility and build. Even cultural differences can come into play. Kneeling and sitting on the heels, for example, might be considered extreme flexion by some, but in the Far East it is part of the normal range of movements. In Japan, you kneel to eat. Squatting down is also often considered extreme flexion, but again in the Far East it is a common position in daily activities, including both working and eating. Kneeling and bowing down to the floor is a prayer position for Muslims, just as sitting cross-legged is in Buddhism.

Personal judgement is needed. I tend to disagree with the current trend in sports science to consider any position that requires "extreme flexion" to be unsafe. Nevertheless, there are instances, as I explain below, when extreme flexion is dangerous. Generally speaking, if you experience pain and discomfort, it is not for you. In this context, stretching is inadvisable for anyone who has an injured joint, however "safe" the position. Wait until you are fully recovered.

Always stretch when the muscles are warm and not before. Stretching involves the opening of joints to a greater angle than in regular activity. This has to be done slowly and without force. Ball and socket joints are especially unstable. Excessive straightening of hinge joints, such as the knee, can also cause stress and damage. Practice breathing slowly and evenly to relax the muscles, because quick and excitable breathing tenses up the muscles. It is also important to bring the synergistic muscles into play to help stabilize joints and support the stretches. The instructions presented throughout the rest of this chapter are as important as the illustrations, because they take you stage by stage through the stretch. Give yourself ample space in which to work, and do not hurry the exercises. (Appendix 3 provides suggestions on how to sequence the different stretch exercises.)

I have divided the stretches into those for the torso, the upper limbs, and the lower limbs. In the instructions, I have emphasized the technique of breathing with the diaphragm to improve balance, control, and muscle relaxation. The instruction to inhale means breathing in deeply to let the diaphragm and the abdomen move, allowing the maximum expansion of the lungs; the instruction to exhale means breathing out to let the stomach muscles return closer to the back of the spine. In stretching, exhalation should be slow and controlled and not as strong as in muscular strength-training exercises. Finally, **breathe normally when you are holding a stretch.**

The Torso

Back Muscles: Erector Spinae, Transversospinalis-Multifidus, Trapezius, and Latissimus Dorsi

Feline Stretch (Erector Spinae)

- Kneel on the floor, making sure that the hips are aligned above the knee.

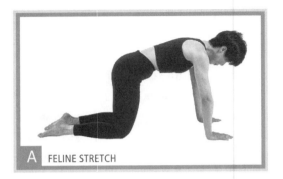

A | FELINE STRETCH

- Place both hands on the floor, directly below the shoulders.

- Keeping the face down, take a deep breath.

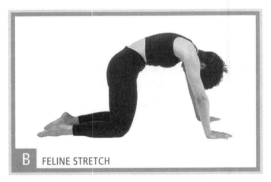

B | FELINE STRETCH

- Exhale, tucking the tummy in, and at the same time tuck in your chin and round the buttocks under. Exhaling enables you to round the back in more of a stretch and also helps support the trunk.

- Hold the stretch for 10 to 12 seconds.

- Gently return the back and neck to their original position. During the movement take care not to hyperextend the neck or let the spine sag into an inverted arch.

- Repeat the stretch two to three times, holding slightly longer in each session.

The feline stretch also lengthens the trapezius muscles, between the shoulder blades (see page 135). If you repeat the stretch two or three times, you should notice an easing of the muscles running from the neck down the back and between the shoulder blades, and a greater relief of tension than if you do just a single long stretch.

Prayer Position (Latissimus Dorsi)

 - Kneel and rest your buttocks on your heels and stretch both arms out in front on the floor. Keep your face and trunk close to the floor and tuck the buttocks well under. This is a good stretch for the latissimus dorsi and back (see page 135).

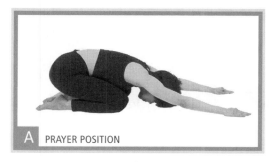

A PRAYER POSITION

Half Serpent (Erector Spinae, Transversospinalis-Multifidus, and Latissimus Dorsi)

The half serpent mobilizes the vertebrae and lengthens the back muscles. This is an advanced position and should be attempted only after the feline and prayer positions have been mastered.

- Start from the prayer position.

- Take a deep breath and then exhale, keeping the tummy tucked in.

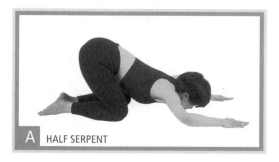

A HALF SERPENT

- Breathing normally, glide forward with the chin and chest close to the floor until the head is between the palms of the hands.

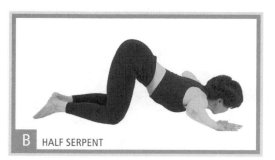

B HALF SERPENT

- Inhale and come up in a feline stretch, arms fully extended (see A, page 148).

- Exhale and tuck your head down, keeping the back rounded and the bottom tucked under (see B, page 148). Hold.

- Release and return to the prayer position. The movement should be slow and controlled, with even breathing.

- Repeat two to three times.

This is a wonderful, safe stretch that helps mobilize the joints between the vertebrae. You should feel slight movements in them as you glide forward. With practice your movements should become graceful and you should feel a strengthening and lengthening of the spinal muscles. Your ability to turn and twist will improve.

Full Serpent (Erector Spinae and Latissimus Dorsi)

This advanced position is not suitable for people with weak back or tummy muscles. Based on yoga, it can be a dangerous stretch if you let the small of the back pinch inward. Carefully following the step-by-step instructions avoids this.

- Start from the prayer position (see page 149). Keep your face and trunk close to the floor and tuck your buttocks well under. Keep the tummy tight.

- Breathing normally, glide forward, keeping the chin and chest close to the floor, until your head moves past your hands and the body is almost completely prone.

- On the next out-breath, tilt the pelvis slightly forward so that the pubic bone touches the floor. The pelvic tilt stops the small of the back from sagging and pinching inward.

- Breathe in and exhale while you lift the body, coming to rest on your elbows.

- Hold.

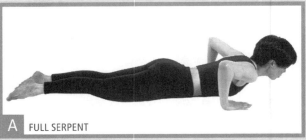

A FULL SERPENT

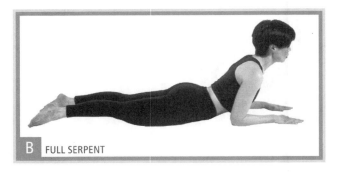

B FULL SERPENT

- Release, breathing out and gliding back to the prayer position.

An alternative advanced finish, called the *full cobra*, is recommended only if you have mastered full pelvic and transverse abdominal control. Well executed, however, it is a good back-extension exercise that helps maintain lower-back mobility. Instead of resting on the elbows, place the hands on the floor on either side of the chest, fingers pointing forward. Now push upward on your hands to raise the upper torso, extending the arms fully. Make sure that your head is facing forward. Do

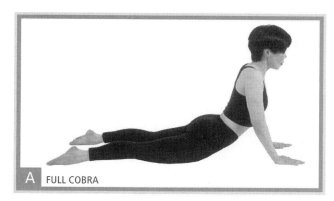

A | FULL COBRA

not tilt the head backward, because that will hyperextend the neck. You should not feel any stress in your lower back if the tummy is tightly controlled and the pubic bone is firmly on the floor. The hamstring will tighten where it meets the buttock.

Abdominal Muscles: Rectus Abdominus, Transverse Abdominus, and Obliques

The Yawn (Abdominal Muscles and Others)

This is an overall stretch for major muscle groups, including those in the arms, torso, and legs.

- Lie on your back and bring both arms above the head.

- Inhale deeply and stretch out your arms and legs in opposite directions—as though you are going to yawn—until you feel a stretch in the rectus abdominus, the central panel in the stomach area between the sternum and the pubic bone.

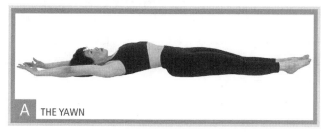

A | THE YAWN

- Hold, breathing normally.

- Exhale and release.

"Z" Stretch (Obliques)

 - Lie on your back, drawing up your knees and keeping your feet flat on the floor.

- Exhale, and, keeping the knees close together, gently lower them to one side of your body. At the same time, rotate the trunk toward the opposite side.

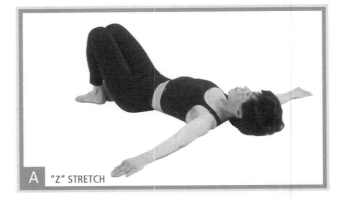

A "Z" STRETCH

- The arms can be extended out from the shoulders in both directions, keeping the shoulders on the floor. Alternatively, point both arms in the direction opposite the knees. The first arm position is more difficult and advanced.

- Hold the position, breathing evenly.

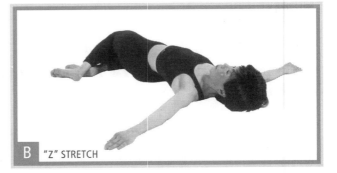

B "Z" STRETCH

- Exhale and release by bringing the knees up to the original position. Repeat on the opposite side.

The movements should be slow and controlled. Care should be taken not to drop the knees abruptly to the floor. Those with back problems or the elderly should use a rolled towel or flat cushion to support the knees when they are brought down to the side, so that the angle of the knee drop, and therefore the stretch of the obliques, is reduced. This stretch incorporates a moderate spinal twist, which is also beneficial for the back.

Chest/Back Muscles: Pectoralis, Trapezius, and Latissimus Dorsi

The Roll-Back (Pectoralis)

Stretching the rectus abdominus in the "yawn" also allows for a slight stretching of the pectoralis because the arms were stretched upwards. This is an additional, more specific stretch for the pectoralis, which can be done either standing up or seated cross-legged.

- Bring both arms to the back, clasp the hands together, and inhale.

- Hold.

- Exhale to release, bringing the hands to their normal position.

Whether standing or sitting, hold the tummy in to support the back. Do not arch the back or push the buttocks backwards.

The Roll-Forward (Trapezius and Latissimus Dorsi)

- Stand or sit cross-legged, keeping the body tall.

- Inhale, and then exhale to let the navel sink toward the spine.

- Breathing normally, bring both arms forward, slightly above shoulder height, to clasp your hands. The shoulders are rounded forward in this motion until a stretch is felt in the muscles between the shoulder blade (trapezius) and those running below the arms to the spine (the latissimus dorsi). Keep the head inclined slightly forward. This helps lengthen the whole of the spinal column.

- Hold and then release.

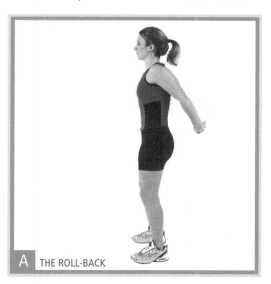

A — THE ROLL-BACK

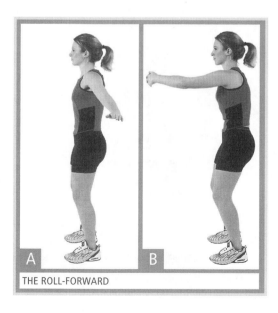

A — B — THE ROLL-FORWARD

This is a wonderful stretch for releasing tension in the trapezius and even the rhomboids. Both muscles act as a brace to hold the shoulders, and they become tense if a lot of time is spent sitting at a desk.

Forearm Twist (Trapezius, Latissimus Dorsi, and Deltoids)

- Stand or sit cross-legged, keeping the body tall.

- Place your hands on the opposite shoulders so that one elbow is resting in the crook of the other arm.

- Bring the forearms together in front of your face, with the palms of the hands facing each other. Bring the palms as closely together as possible, keeping the elbows in place.

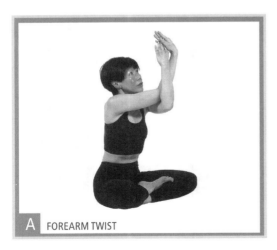

A FOREARM TWIST

- Inhale, raising the arms so that the elbows are about level with your mouth or until you feel a stretch in the muscles between the shoulder blades.

- Exhale, bringing the forearms down again to around chest level so that the upper arms are parallel to the floor. The stretch in the trapezius muscle should intensify.

- Hold, breathing normally, and then release.

The Arms

Biceps, Triceps, and Deltoids

Stretching these muscles has already been covered in Chapter 6 (see page 73). The same exercises, but held longer, can be used for the final stretch.

The Buttocks and Legs

Abductors, Gluteals, and Tensor Fascia Latae

Buttocks Stretch (Gluteals and Tensor Fascia Latae)

- Lie on your back with your knees drawn up and feet firmly placed on the floor. Breathe normally.

- Bring one foot up to rest the ankle on the opposite knee. The knee of the lifted leg will be turned out to the side.

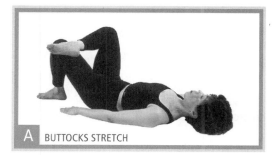

A BUTTOCKS STRETCH

 ■ In the next out-breath, raise the supporting leg off the floor, bringing the supporting knee towards you, until a stretch is felt on the gluteals and the outer thigh area (tensor fascia latae) of the opposite leg (see page 115).

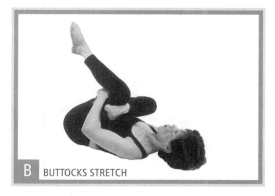

B BUTTOCKS STRETCH

■ Hold, breathing normally, and then gently release.

■ Repeat, using the opposite leg.

It is important to exhale when you raise your legs toward you so that the hip joints are stabilized by the transverse abdominus, which contracts to hold the lower torso in place. The movements should be slow and controlled.

Hold the Horns (Gluteals, Tensor Fascia Latae)

This is an alternative hip stretch.

■ Lie on your back with both legs up in the air, so that the feet are directly above the hips. The knees should be slightly bent.

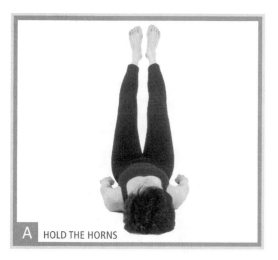

A HOLD THE HORNS

■ Exhale as you cross the knees.

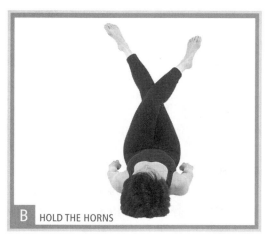

B HOLD THE HORNS

- Grasp the ankles with the hands, bringing the legs further across each other. Keep the knees stacked together. Hold the position, supporting the ankles with the hands and breathing evenly.

 - Inhale, and then as you exhale gently ease the knees closer to the chest, maintaining support of the ankles. When easing the knees toward the chest, try as far as possible to keep the back and hips on the floor. Hold for slightly longer.

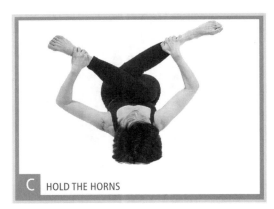

C HOLD THE HORNS

- Repeat by crossing the knees in the opposite direction.

You should feel a stretch in the gluteals and the tensor fascia latae of the top leg.

Adductors

This group of muscles (see illustration on page 122) must be stretched well, largely because they are prone to adaptive shortening. At the end of a workout a developmental stretch should be applied, holding the muscles longer and stretching them more intensely than is necessary for other stretches. This stretch can be done in several ways.

Groin Stretch (Adductors)

- Sit up tall and bring the soles of your feet together. The knees are turned out in opposite directions.

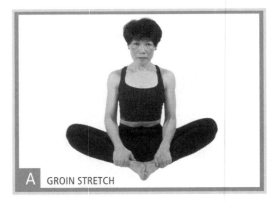

A GROIN STRETCH

- Breathe in, drawing the feet toward the groin, and then exhale gently, easing the knees towards the floor until a stretch is felt in the inner thigh.

- Hold, breathing normally, and then release.

There should be no force exerted on the hip joint. The shoulders should be relaxed and the back straight.

Wide-angle Stretch (Adductors)

- Sit up tall and spread your legs as wide as possible. Take care to ensure that the knees are not turned in but rather are facing upward.

- Breathe in, and then exhale to hold the tummy in and stabilize the hip joint. It's tempting in this position to allow the back to release and curve out behind you; counteract this tendency by using your abdominal muscles to keep the torso tall.

 - On the next out-breath, gently lower the body to the front until a stretch is felt in the inner thigh. Bend forward from the hips; do not allow the torso to collapse. Breathe evenly. Avoid applying any force.

- When the tension of this initial stretch eases, develop the stretch by reaching out further and holding for another 20 to 25 seconds. Exhale as you reach out, but breathe evenly during the stretch. At no point should you hold your breath. If you are very flexible, you could lower your trunk all the way to the floor, developing the stretch into one for the muscles in the back. More will be said about this later in the chapter (see page 160).

The Thigh, Shin, and Calf Muscles

Quadriceps and Tibialis Anterior

Thigh and Shin-muscle Stretch (Quadriceps and Tibialis Anterior)

- Lie face down with your legs fully extended. Keep the knees together.

- On the next out-breath, tilt the pelvis forward until the pubic bone is on the floor.

- Breathing normally, bring one foot toward the buttocks and grasp the foot

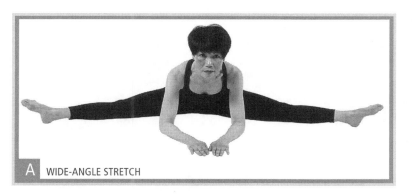

A WIDE-ANGLE STRETCH

with the hand. Pointing the toes of the bent leg will increase the stretch in the quadriceps and stretch the muscle in the shin (the tibialis anterior).

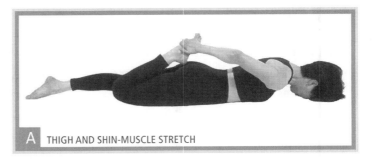

A THIGH AND SHIN-MUSCLE STRETCH

- Hold and then release.

This stretch can also be done standing up or lying on the side.

Hamstring

Examples of how to stretch the hamstring have already been provided earlier in this chapter and in the section on preparatory stretches in Chapter 6. The hamstring needs developmental stretches at the end of activities because it is prone to adaptive shortening. Any of the methods illustrated previously (see exercises on pages 145–146) could be used. However, to turn these into developmental stretches, hold the initial stretch until the tension eases, and then take the stretch slightly further without force, holding for 20–25 seconds more. One additional, advanced hamstring stretch is as follows.

Forward-Bend Stretch (Hamstring)

A ▪ Sit up tall with both legs extended in front.

▪ Inhale, lifting the upper torso tall.

B ▪ Exhale, letting the navel sink toward the spine and keeping the tummy tucked in tight. Lean forward, reaching for your toes until you feel a

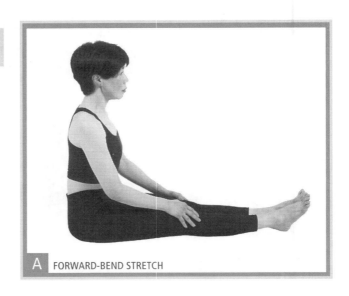

A FORWARD-BEND STRETCH

stretch in the hamstring. Breathe normally. If the feet are flexed, you will also stretch the gastrocnemius (calves). The flexion of the feet should be supported by the hands.

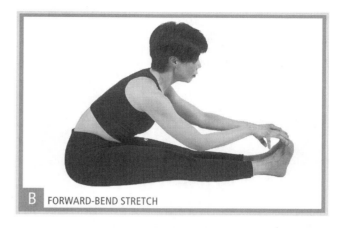

 ▪ Hold until the tightness eases, and then try to reach further toward the toes to develop the stretch.

B FORWARD-BEND STRETCH

The extent to which the upper trunk can move forward varies widely. The trunk of very flexible people may well touch the legs, allowing the hands to grasp the feet. This finishing position is considered extreme flexion, but for the very supple the hamstrings cannot be

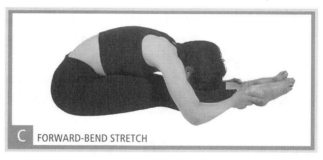

C FORWARD-BEND STRETCH

stretched thoroughly without it. There should be no pain in the hamstrings or stress in the back if full abdominal control is mastered.

Alternatively, instead of stretching both legs at the same time, you can stretch each in turn by bending the resting leg and placing its heel close to the groin or knee of the straightened leg. Continue as above.

Calf Muscle: Gastrocnemius

Examples of how to stretch the gastrocnemius, the calf muscle, have already been given in the sections discussing active and externally assisted stretching of the hamstrings and the forward-bend stretch. The gastrocnemius is another muscle that should be stretched for longer than usual because it is subject to continuous activity and contraction. Stretching this muscle will help reduce soreness and muscle bulk. If the gastrocnemius is stretched by actively flexing the foot, then instead of developing the stretch through long holds, repeat the stretch. Otherwise, as explained previously, the opposing muscle group—the tibialis anterior in this case—will be stressed, because it is the muscle that helps flex the foot.

Progression in Training

Full Wide-angle Stretch (Adductors, Erector Spinae, and Latissimus Dorsi)

Once muscles gain, or regain, their suppleness, the stretch positions described above can be taken further. Consider, for example, the wide-angle stretch, for the adductors. The angle, and thus the stretch, can be widened by spreading the legs further apart (see photo below). The intensity of the stretch can also be increased by reaching out further to the front and making greater use of the floor by stretching the adductors against it. The aim is to lengthen the body forward while avoiding a downward curve in the neck and upper back that would exert

pressure on the cervical spine. The neck must be kept relaxed. Strong abdominal-muscle control prevents the hips from rolling forward. The exercise incorporates a stretch on the erector spinae and the latissimus dorsi. The length of time for which the stretch is held can also be increased slightly.

The full wide-angle stretch represents a progression in flexibility training that keeps the basic stretch position unchanged, but modifies the intensity and angle of stretch. Eventually, you might be able to reach out until your chest is on the floor, but then again you might not! It presents a goal to work towards, but it is not an end in itself. For those who can bring their chest to the floor without any strain, holding the body midway to the ground, rather than lowering it all the way, creates a contrary exercise involving isometric contraction to hold the trunk up. This is where the physiological and physical differences between people

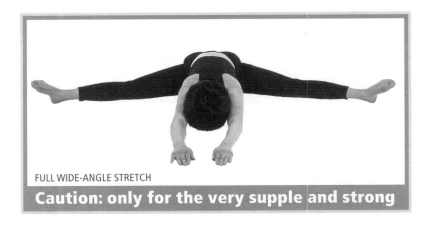

FULL WIDE-ANGLE STRETCH

Caution: only for the very supple and strong

must be recognized and stretches adapted to suit the individual.

Stretching in Flight (Hamstring and Gastrocnemius)

This is an advanced stretch used for both the hamstring and the gastrocnemius.

- Sit up tall in the cross-legged position.

- Inhale, lifting the torso, and then exhale, tucking the navel toward the spine. Breathe evenly.

- Keeping your back straight, draw one knee close to the chest. Now slowly extend or straighten the leg, pointing the toes toward the ceiling, exhaling in the process.

- Hold the leg with both hands to support it. You should feel a strong stretch at the back of the leg, running from the hamstring down to the calves.

- Let the stretch settle; now gently bend the knee to bring it even closer to the body, and straighten the leg again. You should feel a stronger stretch.

- Release and repeat with the other leg.

The closer you can bring your leg toward you and the straighter the leg, the stronger the stretch. But do not use force. For many, the leg will be extended at an angle to the front rather than upward. Apart from its direct impact on the hamstring and gastrocnemius, this stretch also helps improve coordination and balance.

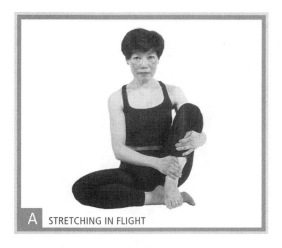

A STRETCHING IN FLIGHT

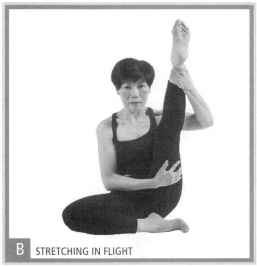

B STRETCHING IN FLIGHT

Full Flight

People who are very strong can stretch both legs upward simultaneously, supported with both hands. This stretch should be attempted only if you have good control over your abdominal muscles and a sound grasp of the technique for stabilizing the hip joint. **Caution: This exercise is only for the very supple and strong.**

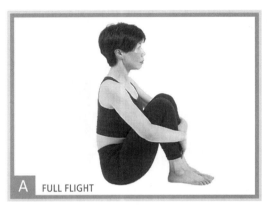

A FULL FLIGHT

 A · Sit up tall.

B · Inhale and draw both knees close to the chest.

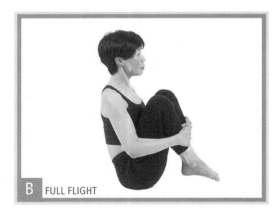

B FULL FLIGHT

C · Exhale, and straighten both legs, pointing them towards the ceiling. Support both legs with the hands, breathing normally.

Breathe evenly while holding the stretch, but do not lean heavily backward or round the back, because this will pass the stress to the small of the back. Do not attempt this advanced stretch if you have back problems. If at any point you are uncomfortable, abandon the stretch.

The progression in flexibility training can also involve adopting even more extreme stretch positions. For example, the

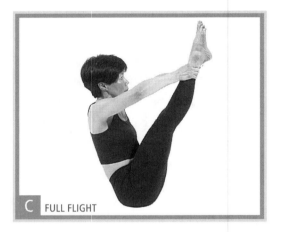

C FULL FLIGHT

plow position, described in Chapter 5, is used to lengthen the erector spinae. It is not recommended for general use and has in fact been deemed dangerous. I must confess that I do occasionally practice the plow, a stretch with which I have had a love–hate relationship for some 20 years, having been taught it long before I realized the dangers associated with its practice. Like an alcoholic returning to the bottle, I return to doing it as a test of my flexibility. Unless you have practiced it since you were young or have previous training in dance, ballet, or gymnastics, the plow carries risks that might not be worth taking. Many other stretches exist that are equally effective for the erector spinae. The general recommendation for flexibility training is to opt for alternative, safer methods.

Overstretching the ligaments can result in instability in the joints. Ligaments, once stretched, remain stretched because they are tough, fibrous tissues. It is for this reason that expectant mothers are advised not to take advantage of the hormone relaxin circulating in their system, which provides increased flexibility, to stretch more intensely than they could do normally. When the hormone level declines after pregnancy, the hip joint in particular becomes unstable if it has been overstretched. The damage may not be apparent when the woman is young, but it can come to light when her muscles weaken with age. The problems related to stretching are dealt with in more detail in Chapter 11.

Relaxation

We have now come to the end of the workout. This is the time to complete the cycle of exercises by allowing the muscles to relax and the body to savor the release in tension that comes after the stretch.

I always like to work with music. For this segment of the workout choose music that is calm and soothing and let it wash over you.

Lying Down

You can lie down on your back, palms turned up to face the ceiling, feet either drawn up or fully extended in front of you, whichever way feels more comfortable. Make sure that your body is aligned. Close your eyes and breathe evenly and slowly, turning your head from side to side to release the tension in the neck. Relax the forehead, relax the jaw, and let the body feel heavy on the floor. Release the shoulders and feel their weight on the floor. Lie quietly and continue to breathe evenly.

When you are ready, stretch both arms on the floor straight above your head. Hold the stretch and then release. Repeat. Stay quiet for a couple more minutes and then gently roll up.

Adaptation of Qi Gong Breathing Technique

Here's a technique I find extremely calming. I have adapted it to make it a pelvic-floor exercise as well as a relaxation technique. Hence, this is not exactly how a qi gong kung fu si fu (master of qi gong) would perform the exercise, which in the original version relates breathing to acupressure points for self-healing.

Sit cross-legged, with the palms of the hand turned up on each knee and the thumb touching the third finger to make a circle. Look downward, but don't allow your head to simply flop forward. Check that the weight of your body is evenly distributed on both sides of your bottom. Close your eyes. Start by breathing evenly.

Now imagine that there's a little steel marble at the base of your body and that your body is generating a magnetic field. Contract the pelvic floor, begin inhaling in a long, slow breath, and imagine drawing the marble up the front of your body, all the way up your abdomen, neck, chin, nose, and forehead, to the top of your skull. Then exhale, long and slowly, imagining the marble rolling gently down your back.

As you breathe in, curl the tongue backward along the upper palate of the mouth; at the same time, tilt the head upward until the eyes, if they were open, would be reverted at an angle toward the ceiling (you should not tilt your head back fully). On the out-breath, unfurl the tongue, slowly and gently lowering the head until it is again in the starting position.

Repeat this breathing process at least 10 times, and feel the tension release from your body. Then revert back to even breathing. When you are ready, gently open your eyes and stand up.

11

Sports and Exercise Injuries and Training to Avoid Them

All activities carry some risk, even crossing the road. Sports and exercise are no exception. It is estimated that over 10 million sports injuries occur each year. Many of them are a result of accidents, but a significant proportion are from repetitive stresses and strains on joints, muscles, tendons, and ligaments. These can occur as a result of overuse or overtraining, wrong techniques, poor equipment, or even unbalanced muscle development. This chapter reviews some of the more common injuries, their causes, and how they might be avoided.

Common Sports Injuries

Sports injuries come in a variety of forms, depending on the cause of the damage.

- *Sprains* are caused by sudden twists or wrenches of the joints, especially the ankles, knees, or wrists.

- *Strains* result from force, overuse, and overstretching muscles or tendons.

- *Contusions* are caused by a severe blow or force, as when kicked or punched.

- *Fractures* of bones are either simple, compound, or stress/hairline fractures. In simple and compound fractures, the breakage is usually complete; part of the bone may even penetrate through the skin. In stress and hairline fractures, a fine crack runs partially or completely through the bone. Simple and compound fractures are normally caused by the impact of sudden force, whereas hairline fractures are generally associated with overuse and stress.

Injuries to joints are among the most common sports injuries. This is largely because joints bear the brunt of the force applied by muscle contractions against resistance. Although the surfaces of joints are cushioned by cartilage, their resilience deteriorates with continuous use. Wear and tear of or damage to the cartilage causes the opposing surfaces of the joints to roughen and grate against each other, making the joint prone to arthritis and bursitis. Arthritis—that is, inflammation of a joint—results in pain, stiffness, and swelling. In bursitis, the bursa, a fluid-filled sac that surrounds the joint, becomes inflamed, resulting in pain.

When joints are subjected to large force, they can get twisted out of position.

People who play sports that involve sudden changes in direction and acceleration, such as soccer, squash, and tennis, are prone to knee injuries.

Incorrect training that results in or encourages imbalanced development of the quadriceps can cause a misalignment of the patella or kneecap, sometimes referred to as "runner's knee." Wrong technique in leg-extension exercises, especially if external weights are used or if exercises are carried out incorrectly using a machine, is another cause of knee injuries.

Bone injuries include stress fractures such as shin splints. Overuse and overtraining are usually the main causes, aided and abetted by weight-bearing activities such as running on hard surfaces while wearing footwear that provides inadequate cushioning for the force sustained by the lower leg, especially the tibia and toes. Poor biomechanics (flat or highly arched feet, or an abnormal gait) and styles of running can also cause shin splints. Repeated stress on the foot can result in a benign growth of bone, called a *spur*, which can be intensely painful. For example, continued stress on the heel bone can result in calcification of the ligaments originating from it, causing a spur to form at the insertion of the Achilles tendon.

Muscle injuries are common. They range from bruises, resulting from external forces that rupture small blood vessels, to cramps and spasms as a result of inadequate warm-up, dehydration, or fatigue. Injuries can also result from a rekindling of previous damage, such as strains or muscle tear, due to overtraining or overstretching. A sudden contraction of the hamstring, especially following inadequate warm-up and preparatory stretching, can result in a torn or pulled muscle. A pulled muscle can also be caused by any imbalances in muscle strength, for example, very strong quadriceps and relatively weak hamstrings. Muscle injuries can also arise when movement is constrained by tightness in the joints. The inability of the hip joint to open up to its full range of movement can tear the adductor muscles when unexpectedly wide movements are made with the leg.

Tendon injuries, in contrast to muscle injuries, are relatively rare, although they can be very serious and painful. Tendons can be ruptured or become inflamed, resulting in tendonitis. Overuse, exercise on uneven terrain, and tight tendons are possible causes for the rupture of the Achilles tendon. The Achilles tendon is a strong fibrous tissue that connects the gastrocnemius, the muscle in the back of the lower leg, to the heel bone. Abrupt footwork and repeated stress can cause the tendon to snap (see below). Stretching the calf muscles and Achilles tendon helps prevent this.

Poor training and biomechanics can cause inflammation of the iliotibial band, the group of fibrous tissues that connects the gluteal muscles and the tensor fascia

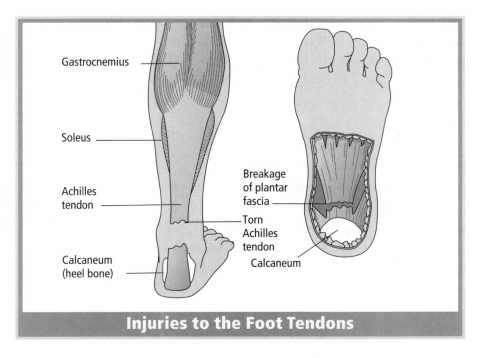

Injuries to the Foot Tendons

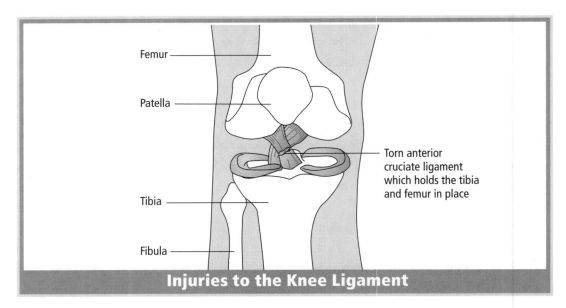

Femur

Patella

Torn anterior cruciate ligament which holds the tibia and femur in place

Tibia

Fibula

Injuries to the Knee Ligament

lata muscle to the tibia, just below the knee. This manifests itself in a pain in the lower outer thigh or the side of the knee. A common cause of this injury is running on only one side of cambered roads. The slope creates a sideways tilt in the pelvis, causing consistent stress to the iliotibial band. Unbalanced muscles, such as tight gluteals or quadriceps, can make the situation worse (see pages 142–143).

Ligaments can be injured, but the symptoms are often manifested in the form of joint pains or joint instability, because ligaments join bone to bone. Ligaments do not heal easily. An extreme example of a ligament injury is when it becomes overstressed and snaps. The anterior cruciate ligaments (see illustration above) are located in the center of the knee, running

from the back of the femur to the front of the tibia. They function as a stabilizer, holding the tibia and femur in place. If excessive force is applied when the knee is bent, the ligament can be injured. In extreme cases, the ligament may tear and snap. The result is a fall and extreme pain and swelling around the knee.

Safe Training

In any discussion of the topic, repeated stress and overtraining emerge as major factors in sports injuries. Poor biomechanics, poor training methods, the wrong use of equipment (including inappropriate footwear), and muscular imbalance are among the others. The principles of good training address these major areas, most of which

Selected Major Sports and Exercise Injuries

Location	Problem	Symptoms	Causes	Prevention
Joints	Arthritis (most forms are not a direct result of sports injuries, e.g., rheumatoid, seronegative, infective, ankylosing spondylitis, gout)	Inflammation, pain, stiffness	Cartilage damage (causes unrelated to sports injury are not covered here)	None, but keeping joints mobile and adopting a cautious approach to loaded and repetitive movements help minimize cartilage damage
	Synovitis	Inflammation of the synovial membrane, local swelling, tenderness, and pain	Local trauma, arthritis, overuse, infection	Cautious approach to loaded and repe-titive movements
	Baker's cyst	Painless fluid-filled swelling behind knee	Torn cartilage, weakness of knee capsule, arthritis	Cautious approach to loaded and repetitive movement
	Runner's knee, or chondromalacia patellae	Acute knee pain	Quadriceps imbalance, sustained damage, poor biomechanics	Improvement of muscle balance and strength, proper footwear
	Bursitis, e.g. housemaid's knee (prepatellar bursitis), clergyman's knee (tibial tubercle bursitis), tennis elbow (olecranon bursitis), frozen shoulder (can result from deltoid bursitis)	Pain and tenderness, inflammation and swelling from accumulation of fluid	Overuse, direct force, arthritis	Good warm-up and preparatory stretches to help prepare joint
	Ankle sprain	Pain, bruising, swelling	Twisting of ankle	Improvement of joint mobility and strength, proper footwear

(Source: The British Medical Association. *Complete Family Health Encyclopaedia*. London: Dorling Kindersley, 1996; Troop, N., Seato, S. *Handbook of Running*. London: Pelham Books, 1997.)

Selected Major Sports and Exercise Injuries (cont'd.)

Location	Problem	Symptoms	Causes	Prevention
Joints (cont'd.)	Back pain	Pain and reduced mobility	Weak abdominal muscles, poor posture, poor training, excess weight	Improvement of abdominal muscle strength, stretching, proper footwear
Bones	Stress fracture, e.g., shin splints	Pain	Overuse, over-pronation, ill-fitting shoes	Moderate training program, gradual increase in intensity of effort
	Spurs	Benign growth in bone, pain, and inflammation	Repeated stress	Moderate training program, gradual increase in intensity of effort
Muscles	Hamstring pull	Pain, muscle spasm, loss of strength	Sudden contraction of hamstring, overuse of muscle, weak hamstrings relative to quadriceps	Warm-up and stretching before and after activity
	Quadriceps strain/tear	Sudden pain (especially when bending the knee while performing a squat or sitting down), swelling, and tenderness	Sudden contraction of quadriceps, overuse of muscle	Warm-up and stretching before and after activity
	Gastrocnemius strain	Pain (especially when going down the stairs or down a slope), difficulty in supporting body weight	Overuse and over-load of muscle	Warm-up and stretching before and after activity
	Adductor strain/tear	Pain	Overstretching, limited hip mobility	Warm-up and stretching before and after activity

		Selected Major Sports and Exercise Injuries (cont'd.)		
Location	Problem	Symptoms	Causes	Prevention
Tendons	Tendonitis, e.g., Achilles tendonitis	Painful swelling in tendon, sometimes restricted use of muscle to which tendon is connected	Injury; repeated stress and over-load; poor biome-chanics	Moderate training program, proper footwear in case of Achilles tendon
	Rupture, e.g., Achilles tendon rupture	Sudden pain, shock, and swelling; inability to support muscle and weight, immo-bilization	Violent stretching, aggressive stop-and-start footwork, repeated stress	Moderate training program, proper footwear in case of Achilles tendon
	Iliotibial-band friction	Pain in outer knee or lower thigh	Incorrect training, poor biomechanics	Balanced muscle development and training, stretching
Ligaments	Rupture or tear, e.g., anterior cruci-ate ligament	Knee joint sud-denly fails	Excessive force and stress on knee in bent position	Correct training technique and po-sition, avoidance of excessive flexion and force on joints

have already been covered elsewhere in the book.

Moderation is essential in exercise. The body needs adequate rest in order to recover from exertion and to perform well. Exhaustion results in poor coordination, poor performance, and injuries. The principle of overload involves building up greater endurance and strength by progressively giving the body more than its normal workload. This prompts the skeletal muscles, both fast- and slow-twitch, to adapt and develop.

They can only do so, however, if the muscles are not injured or overused. Rest days are essential. It takes the body about 24 hours to restore glycogen levels, the primary source of energy for working muscles (see Chapter 3).

It is important to ensure that the movements that constitute the exercise or sport are executed well. Special attention should be paid to joints, because they take the bulk of the force. Keeping the knees soft when landing after a jump is essential to reduce impact on the knees. Athletes need to be aware of how they walk and run to ensure that their feet land correctly. In running, the heel strikes the ground, the arch flattens to absorb some of the impact, and then the foot rolls inward, allowing the ball of the foot to touch the ground while the heel lifts up. This inward-rolling motion, called *pronation*, allows the push to move forward and helps absorb the shock of landing. Flat feet tend to *overpronate*, that is, to roll inward excessively, causing injuries to the lower leg. High arches in the feet can lead to *underpronation*, causing the ankle to take the shock. Correct footwear can reduce these problems. It is also important not to land on the toes or the ball of the foot when running.

The hip joint and the small of the back, especially the fifth lumbar, are subjected to considerable pressure and stress in some floor exercises. In abdominal curl-ups, for example, it is important to ensure that the small of the back is supported and not arched. Stabilize the hips by drawing the knees up and engaging the iliopsoas muscle to act as a synergist muscle. Correct breathing and engagement of the transverse abdominus, two practices I have repeatedly stressed in this book, contribute greatly to a safer and more effective workout.

Excessive flexion presents another problem. For example, when lunging forward on one leg to stretch the leg extended behind, it is important to align the knee of the front leg above the ankle. If the knee goes beyond the ankle, the entire weight is shifted toward the front and excessive pressure is exerted on the knee and ankle. Dropping the buttocks below knee level when doing squats can be another cause of extreme flexion. The figures below and on the next page provide examples of poor movements and positions that can injure joints.

In floor push-ups (see illustrations on the next page), poor alignment of arms and inadequate stomach control can cause lower-back and shoulder injuries. In "V" sit-ups (see illustration on the next page), employing excessive leverage when raising the trunk stresses the lower back. Frequently, people raise their body by pushing out the stomach muscles, which over time leads to the development of bulging stomach muscles.

It is important to warm up and stretch before and after the completion of an ac-

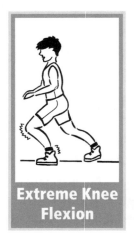

Extreme Knee Flexion

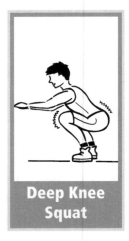

Deep Knee Squat

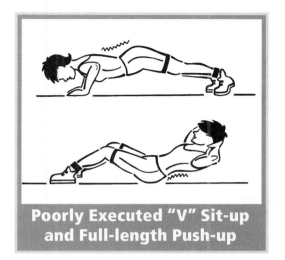

Poorly Executed "V" Sit-up and Full-length Push-up

tivity. Stretching before the activity helps improve performance by loosening the muscles and stretching the tissues of the connective fibers. Reduced muscle tightness decreases the incidence of muscle strain and tear.

Balanced muscle development is extremely important because any imbalance can injure a weaker opposing-muscle group. Shin splints are often caused by a weak tibialis anterior relative to a strong gastrocnemius; hamstring pulls can result from overdeveloped quadriceps; and weak abdominal muscles pass all the effort of body support to the back, stressing the erector spinae. Cross-training is useful in balancing muscle development, especially when a sport or exercise discipline focuses on particular muscle groups or on a limited range of the five principles of fitness (see Chapter 2 for a discussion of these).

When training to develop muscular strength and endurance, the movements should be slow and controlled. Avoid large or vigorous movements. When stretching, avoid ballistic stretches. The body should be taken to its natural joint range, but extreme movements that cause discomfort and pain should be avoided.

Treatment for Sports Injuries

The recommended first aid for all injuries, including strains, sprains, and fractures, is indicated by the acronym RICE. This stands for **R**est, application of **I**ce, **C**ompression, and **E**levation of the injured part above the level of the heart. Rest or ceasing the activity helps prevent further damage; ice helps reduce bleeding and swelling; compression reduces swelling; and elevation assists in the drainage of fluid from the injured part. Do not, however, try to treat your own injuries. Contact a doctor immediately or as soon as possible. A correct diagnosis is essential for prescribing treatment.

12

Nutrition: The Other Side of the Fitness Equation

Achieving the right balance between energy intake and expenditure is of prime importance in weight control. To get the balance correct we might calculate our basic metabolic rate, add an estimate of the amount of energy we expend on day-to-day life, and allow for any extra physical activities or sports (see Chapter 4). But what we eat cannot be limited to calculations of energy; food affects our health and our bodily functions and is tied in with our cultural and social interactions. Great enjoyment is derived from good food combined with good company. We are, in every respect, what we eat.

In this book, however, we will restrict the discussion to the physiological aspects of food and nutrition. In short, we need to balance our nutritional needs as well as our energy requirements. There is a tendency to discount nutritional needs, particularly among women, and to place undue emphasis on body weight and the notion of slimming. This preoccupation has resulted in wave after wave of diets, ranging from high-protein to high-fiber, fruit-and-vegetable-only, no- or low-fat, and even detox diets, where the emphasis seems to be more on starving than eating. Most of these diets will help a person reduce his or her weight, but may bear repercussions on health if followed for long. Moreover, unless good eating habits are developed, the loss in weight is likely to be followed with a vengeance by weight

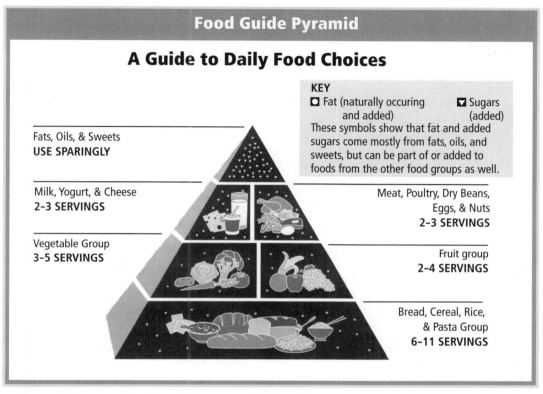

Food Guide Pyramid

A Guide to Daily Food Choices

KEY
◻ Fat (naturally occuring and added)   ☑ Sugars (added)
These symbols show that fat and added sugars come mostly from fats, oils, and sweets, but can be part of or added to foods from the other food groups as well.

Fats, Oils, & Sweets
USE SPARINGLY

Milk, Yogurt, & Cheese
2-3 SERVINGS

Meat, Poultry, Dry Beans, Eggs, & Nuts
2-3 SERVINGS

Vegetable Group
3-5 SERVINGS

Fruit group
2-4 SERVINGS

Bread, Cereal, Rice, & Pasta Group
6-11 SERVINGS

(Source: U.S. Department of Agriculture/U.S. Department of Health and Human Services)

gain once the diet is abandoned. Health is not about thinness. It is about being fit, which means having sufficient energy and nutrition for physical activities *and* a healthy body. So let's put aside fashion and fads and get back to basics.

Balancing Food Requirements

The dietary balance recommended by the World Health Organization for an average person is 55 to 75 percent of calories from carbohydrates, 15 to 30 percent from fat,

and 10 to 15 percent from protein. In addition, we need vitamins, minerals, and water. It is important to note, however, that these are general recommendations. They do not represent targets for individuals, which vary depending on body proportions, weight, height, age, gender, and activity/work. They also vary according to country, based on different cultures' consumption characteristics (see Chapter 4 and page 54). In the United States, for example, the government-recommended guideline for fat intake is no more than 30 percent of calories (with no

What Counts as One Serving?

The amount of food that counts as one serving is listed below. If you eat a larger portion, count it as more than 1 serving. For example, a dinner portion of spaghetti would count as 2 or 3 servings of pasta.

Be sure to eat at least the lowest number of servings from the five major food groups listed below. You need them for the vitamins, minerals, carbohydrates, and protein they provide. Just try to pick the lowest fat choices from the food groups. No specific serving size is given for the fats, oils, and sweets group because the message is USE SPARINGLY.

Milk, Yogurt, and Cheese:
1 cup of milk or yogurt; 1½ ounces of natural cheese; 2 ounces of processed cheese

Meat, Poultry, Fish, Dry Beans, Eggs, and Nuts:
2–3 ounces of cooked lean meat, poultry, or fish; 1–1½ cups of cooked dry beans; 2 eggs; or 4–5 tablespoons of peanut butter

Vegetable:
1 cup of raw leafy vegetables; ½ cup of other vegetables, cooked or raw; ¾ cup of vegetable juice

Fruit:
1 medium apple, banana, orange; ½ cup of chopped, cooked, or canned fruit; ¾ cup of fruit juice

Bread, Cereal, Rice, and Pasta:
1 slice of bread; 1 ounce of ready-to-eat cereal; ½ cup of cooked cereal, rice, or pasta

(Source: www.nal.usda.gov:8001/py/pmap.htm)

more than 10 percent of calories from saturated fat); in the United Kingdom, by contrast, the government has set the maximum recommended fat intake at 35 percent of calories.

The dietary guidelines for healthy eating in the United States are set out in the Food Guide Pyramid (see page 175). Developed as an easy guide for good eating habits, the pyramid emphasizes the importance of a balanced total diet and the eating of many different foods, a view not unlike that of the WHO. The pyramid encourages people to eat larger proportions of foods high in carbohydrates compared to foods high in protein. For example, 6–11 servings of bread, cereal, rice, and pasta are recommended compared to 2–3 servings of the meat, poultry, fish, dry beans, eggs, and nut group and 2–3 servings of dairy products such as milk, yogurt, and cheese. In each food group, a range of servings are recommended to suit people with different recommended total daily allowance of calorie intake. The lower servings of each food group correspond to

Foods Rich in Carbohydrates

Grain sources	Vegetable sources
Wheat Bread (brown, white, whole-grain, multigrain) Pasta and noodles Wheat germ Farina (cream of wheat) Spelt and spelt products Couscous	*Roots and tubers* Potatoes, sweet potatoes, cassava, yams, parsnips, beets, tapioca, Jerusalem artichokes, jicama
Rice Cooked rice (steamed, boiled, fried, paella, risotto, pilaf) Rice products (vermicelli, rice pancakes, rice dumplings, rice cakes)	*Legumes* Beans (kidney beans, black beans, lima beans, navy beans, black-eyed peas, pinto beans), lentils (red and green), chickpeas, peas, sugar snap peas
Maize/corn and hominy Sweet corn (canned, on the cob, creamed) Corn products (cornbread, tortillas, polenta) Hominy (whole, grits)	**Fruit sources** Dried fruits (raisins, currants, dates, prunes) Fresh fruits (apples, bananas, pears, plums, figs, dates, papayas, others)
Oats Oatmeal Oat bran Oat products (oat bread, oat crackers)	**Nuts** Chestnuts (Only the chestnut is listed here because unlike other nuts, which are high in fat and protein, chestnuts are high in carbohydrate and low in protein and fat. Four times more peanuts would be needed to provide the amount of carbohydrate available in the equivalent weight of chestnuts.)
Other grains Breakfast cereals (granola, cornflakes, crisped rice, bran flakes, cereal bars) Bulk grains (quinoa, millet, sorghum, barley, rye)	

those with a total calorie intake of 1,600 or less, while the higher servings of each food group correspond to those with a total calorie intake of 2,800.

What counts as a serving varies with the food concerned. For bread, a slice represents one serving while one serving of cooked cereal is half a cup (see the table on page 176).

Carbohydrates

Carbohydrates consist of starches (complex carbohydrates, or polysaccharides) and sugars (simple carbohydrates, or monosaccharides and disaccharides). Carbohydrates are great providers of energy. All carbohydrates have the same amount of energy: four calories per gram. However, cellulose, the polysaccharide that makes up the bulk of plant cell walls, has no calorie content because it is not digested. Instead it contributes to dietary fiber, which is important for maintaining regular bowel habits. But not all fibers are insoluble. Soluble fiber constituents— e.g., pectin, found in fruits, vegetables, and legumes—are absorbed by the body. Their consumption helps reduce cholesterol in the blood.

Most of our intake of carbohydrate comes from the starch in cereals, flour, bread, potatoes, rice, and pasta. Ideally, complex carbohydrates such as these, rather than sugars, should provide at least 90 percent of the total daily carbohydrate intake. These polysaccharides break up during the process of digestion and are converted by digestive enzymes into the monosaccharide glucose. Glucose is absorbed into the blood for immediate use or is stored either as body fat or in muscle cells and in the liver as glycogen. The glycogen stored in muscle cells converts to glucose for energy release. The glycogen stored in the liver releases glucose to maintain blood sugar levels, ensuring an adequate supply of energy to the brain and nervous system.

The remainder of the carbohydrate intake (between 5 and 10 percent of total calorie intake) should come from sugars in the form of sucrose, lactose, and maltose. During digestion, these simple carbohydrates are broken down and absorbed into the bloodstream for immediate use or storage. Most of the sugar in the typical Western diet is in the form of sucrose, nearly all of which comes from commercially produced white sugar. Refined sugar is considered to be of poor nutritional value because it contains only energy. By contrast, most foods high in complex carbohydrates (polysaccharides) also contain minerals, including iron, and vitamins. A person consuming about 2,200 calories per day should aim for a minimum of about 300 grams of carbohydrate (55 percent).

Fats and Fatty Acids

The fat in food provides the most energy: 9 calories per gram. The term *fat* encompasses separated fats such as butter, lard, oil, drippings, and margarine, the visible fat found in meats, and the invisible fat contained in many foods. For example, about 50 percent of the weight of a peanut comes from fat, about 30 percent of the weight of a piece of chocolate or Cheddar cheese comes from fat, about 8 percent of the weight of a piece of raw liver comes from fat, and about 12 percent of the weight of a piece of lean beef comes from fat.

Fats are chemical compounds that contain fatty acids. There are two broad types of fatty acid: saturated fatty acids and unsaturated fatty acids. Unsaturated fatty acids are in turn divided into monounsaturated and polyunsaturated fatty acids. Animal fats and other fats that are solid at room temperature generally contain more saturated fatty acids. Examples include butter, cheese, lard, palm oil, coconut oil, cream, peanut butter, chocolate, and beef, lamb, and pork fat. Unsaturated fats are liquid at room temperature and are contained in plant and fish oils. Examples include olive oil, fish oils (mackerel, sardines, and salmon), almond oil, avocado oil, and some vegetable cooking oils. However, modern food processing has altered this division between solid and liquid fats, making it more difficult to distinguish saturated from unsaturated fats. Vegetable and fish oils can be solidified by the addition of hydrogen, producing trans-fatty acids. Margarine, for example, is produced by the hydrogenation of vegetable oils. These trans fats, produced as a result of hydrogenation, are not the same as naturally occurring trans fats found in some foods of animal origin. Some research suggests a link between a high consumption of artificial trans fats and heart disease because foods high in trans fatty acids tend to raise blood cholesterol.

Fats consumed in food are broken down by the body into triglycerides, which are released into the bloodstream and are either used immediately for energy or stored as fat in the adipose tissues of the body. The liver also produces triglycerides from carbohydrates and protein. Triglycerides are the main type of fat transported in the body. The adipose tissues can be drawn upon to supply energy between meals. Aside from fat stores, the adipose tissues provide insulation that helps to maintain the body temperature, maintain reserves of fat-soluble vitamins (see the section on vitamins later in the chapter), and help cushion body organs such as the heart, reproductive system, and kidneys.

Not all fatty acids need to be provided through the diet. All but two of them, linoleic acid and alpha-linolenic acid, can be synthesized within the body. Because these two cannot be produced within the body, they are referred to as essential fatty acids (EFAs). Linoleic acid (an omega-6 fatty acid) occurs in large amounts in plants and vegetable oils and in small amounts in some animal fats. Vegetable oils with high concentrations of linoleic acids include safflower, sunflower, soy, and corn oils. Alpha-linolenic acid (an omega-3 fatty acid) is found in plant seed oils and fish oils.

Foods and Their Cholesterol Content

High	Egg yolks, organ meats (brains, heart, liver, kidney), cheese, cream, butter, lard, fatty meats, prawns, sardines, milk chocolate, rich cookies, pastries, and cakes
Moderate	Beef, chicken, lamb, pork, rabbit, turkey, cod, lobster, mackerel, oysters
Low	Low-fat cottage cheese, skim milk, salmon, low-fat yogurt
None	All plant foods: vegetables, cereals, fruits, plant oils (cholesterol is found only in foods from animal sources)

Note: Although palm and coconut oils, as plant oils, do not contain any cholesterol, they are very high in saturated fats.

Foods that Lower Blood Cholesterol

Cereal-based foods	Whole-grain bread, multigrain bread, rye crackers, oatmeal, breakfast cereals containing cooked bran, oat bran
Fruits	Apples, avocados, bananas, pears, oranges, dried fruits (prunes, figs, apricots)
Vegetables	Lettuces and other greens, garlic, onions, beans, celery, corn
Polyunsaturated oils	Corn oil, sunflower oil, soybean oil, peanut oil, safflower oil
Monounsaturated oils	Olive oil, avocados, canola oil

Blood Cholesterol Levels and Their Associated Risk Factors*

Total cholesterol levels	Category
Less than 200 mg/dl†	Desirable
200–239 mg/dl	Borderline high
240 mg/dl and above	High. A person with this level has more than twice the risk of heart disease as someone whose cholesterol is below 200 mg/dl.

* Associated risks of high cholesterol include hypertension, coronary heart disease, angina, atherosclerosis, thrombosis.
† mg/dl = Milligrams per deciliter

The essential fatty acids have numerous functions in the body. For example, they are involved in the functioning of cell membranes and the production of hormones as well as the synthesis of other fatty acids. Their importance makes very low-fat diets inadvisable unless medically prescribed. Such a diet also has the inherent danger of depleting the body of fat-soluble vitamins A, D, E, and K.

Cholesterol

In any consideration of fat and health, a major preoccupation is the role of cholesterol, which, like fat, is classified as a lipid. A high level of cholesterol in the blood is associated with a high risk of coronary heart disease (see table on page 180). Unfortunately, focus on this medical aspect of health has given cholesterol the reputation of being a harmful substance and has led to a great deal of misunderstanding.

Cholesterol is produced in the body as part of its normal metabolism; it is continuously being synthesized and broken down. The body can produce most of the cholesterol it needs; the liver alone can produce up to 1 gram per day. Cholesterol provides rigidity to cell membranes, serving a similar purpose in animal cells to that of cellulose in plant cells, and is an important component of the myelin sheath that surrounds nerve fibers. It is needed to produce hormones such as those involved in the control of inflammation, maintaining blood pressure, and contracting the uterus during labor. Cholesterol is also vital to the development of the brain and vascular system of the fetus. Therefore, far from being harmful, cholesterol in the body is essential for development and health.

Cholesterol is moved around the body in the blood, attached to proteins called *lipoproteins*. Cholesterol carried in low-density lipoproteins is called *LDL cholesterol*; cholesterol carried in high-density lipoproteins is called *HDL cholesterol*.

The low-density lipoproteins carry cholesterol to body tissues where it is used for various metabolic functions, including cell repair and the production of hormones, but in the process it deposits some of the cholesterol in the cell walls (especially those in damaged artery linings), where it can build up as plaque. The resulting chronic "furring" of the arteries, called *atherosclerosis*, interferes with the blood flow, causing stress to the heart and circulatory system. Hence, a high level of LDL cholesterol in the blood indicates a greater risk of heart disease. In view of this, LDL cholesterol is often called "bad" cholesterol.

The high-density lipoprotein, in contrast, removes excess cholesterol from the body cells to the liver, where it is broken down to form bile. The bile passes into the gastrointestinal tract, where the cholesterol-rich bile salts emulsify fats in the food, helping the enzyme lipase to break them down for absorption through the intestinal lining. The bile with its waste products is eventually excreted in the feces (see diagram, page 183). A high level of HDL cholesterol, therefore, helps reduce the risk of coronary heart disease. For this reason, it is often called "good" cholesterol.

This loose reference to "bad" and "good" cholesterol has contributed to the misconception that people can improve the cholesterol composition in their blood by eating more "good" and less "bad" cholesterol, but research has failed to demonstrate a clear link between the consumption of cholesterol in foods and cholesterol levels in the blood. In fact, whether cholesterol is "good" or "bad" is not determined by the cholesterol in the food but by the lipoprotein carrier in the blood—that is, LDL versus HDL. There is strong evidence, however, that the consumption of saturated fat increases blood cholesterol levels. Most authorities on heart disease, such as the American Heart Association, consider it much more important to limit foods rich in saturated fats than to cut down on foods high in cholesterol.

Since most of the cholesterol in the blood is LDL cholesterol, the higher the level of cholesterol in the blood, the greater the risk of higher levels of LDL cholesterol. However, because of the different properties of HDL cholesterol and LDL cholesterol, it is important to look at their relative proportions in the blood, in addition to the level of *total* blood cholesterol, when evaluating personal cholesterol levels. The American Heart Association recommends a level of HDL cholesterol above 60 mg/dl, which is considered protective against heart disease. An HDL level below 40 mg/dl is a major risk factor for heart disease. An LDL level below 100 mg/dl is considered optimal; between

130 and 150 mg/dl is borderline high; and above 160 is high.

In brief, the overall consensus is that fat should be part of a balanced diet, but the consumption of saturated fat should be reduced in favor of polyunsaturated and monounsaturated fats, particularly by individuals suffering from heart diseases or excessively high levels of blood cholesterol.[11] Fish oils are recommended because they contain large amounts of omega-3 fatty acids and are a valuable source of iron and the fat-soluble vitamins A, D, and E. Sunflower oil, corn oil, and other vegetable oils, which are good sources of the omega-6 fatty acid, are also recommended. Unlike saturated fats, these polyunsaturated fats do not encourage the deposition of cholesterol onto the linings of arteries, and some studies have shown that they can reduce cholesterol levels. Monounsaturated fats, found for example in olive oil and canola oil, have a similar beneficial effect. They have also been reported to lower the level of LDL cholesterol without affecting that of the beneficial HDL cholesterol.

Meeting these objectives can be a problem. Saturated fat has become an intrinsic ingredient in many foods. The high fat content of modern-day foods combined with the invisibility of fat makes it difficult to moderate fat intake. A fat consumption within the recommended range of 15 per-

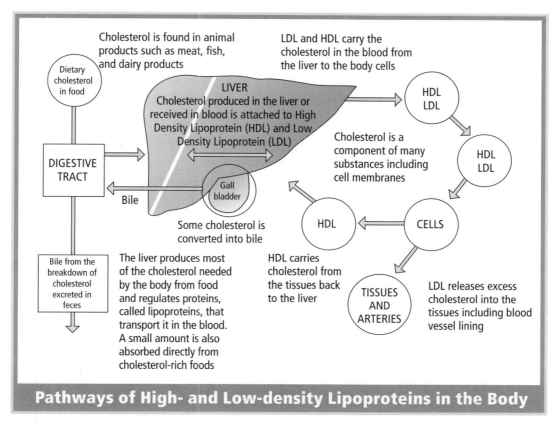

Cholesterol is found in animal products such as meat, fish, and dairy products

LDL and HDL carry the cholesterol in the blood from the liver to the body cells

Dietary cholesterol in food

LIVER
Cholesterol produced in the liver or received in blood is attached to High Density Lipoprotein (HDL) and Low Density Lipoprotein (LDL)

HDL LDL

Cholesterol is a component of many substances including cell membranes

HDL LDL

DIGESTIVE TRACT

Bile

Gall bladder

Some cholesterol is converted into bile

HDL

CELLS

Bile from the breakdown of cholesterol excreted in feces

The liver produces most of the cholesterol needed by the body from food and regulates proteins, called lipoproteins, that transport it in the blood. A small amount is also absorbed directly from cholesterol-rich foods

HDL carries cholesterol from the tissues back to the liver

TISSUES AND ARTERIES

LDL releases excess cholesterol into the tissues including blood vessel lining

Pathways of High- and Low-density Lipoproteins in the Body

cent to 30 percent of total calorie intake seems high, but in practice it is difficult to keep within this limit. Take as an example the average recommended allowance for a woman of 2,200 calories per day. At this calorie level, between 330 and 660 calories could come from fat, equivalent to between 37 and 74 grams of fat. Think of the fat that is in a cookie, a slice of cake, cooking oil, salad dressings, the milk that goes into coffee and tea—the limit is soon reached.

By employing good eating habits based on the Food Guide Pyramid, however, keep-

ing within the 30 percent recommended fat intake can be achieved. By making the effort to choose healthier eating habits, you will make an important step towards overall fitness.

Proteins and Amino Acids

Proteins are essential in our dietary intake because they provide the raw materials for growth and repair and for the production of hormones and enzymes, which regulate cell function. Proteins also provide an emergency source of energy if carbohydrates are in short supply. The name *protein* is derived from a Greek word meaning "first" or "of primary importance." The fact that this nutrient was favored with such a title suggests that its pivotal role in the scheme of life has long been suspected.

To understand the importance of proteins you need only consider the variety of roles they play in the body. Nearly all parts of the body—bones, skin, and muscles—contain collagen, which is a protein. Nails and hair contain the protein keratin, and tendons and arteries contain elastin, another protein. Muscles contain the contractile proteins actin and myosin. In blood, hemoglobin and myoglobin are proteins, as are lipoproteins. Enzymes, the catalysts that make possible the body's complicated biological reactions, are proteins. Proteins also play a prominent part in the body's response to infection, and they help speed recovery. The list of their functions is almost endless.

When proteins in food are digested, they are broken down into the constituent amino acids, which can then be reassembled to provide the proteins needed by the body. The body can also synthesize some amino acids, but not all of them. For adults, eight amino acids, the so-called *essential amino acids*, must be provided from protein in the diet. These eight essential amino acids are isoleucine, leucine, lysine, methio-nine, phenylalanine, threonine; tryptophan, and valine. Children require two additional essential amino acids, arginine and histidine, for growth. Protein from animal food sources contains all the essential amino acids, but plants vary in their content, so vegetarians require a balanced mix of vegetables to meet requirements. Soy is the only plant food that contains all the essential amino acids. Deficiency in protein intake can result in serious disorders such as stunted growth in children, poor muscle development, thin and fragile hair, poor skin quality, and, in cases of severe protein malnutrition in children, *kwashiorkor*.

The term kwashiorkor comes from the Ga dialect of western Africa and means literally "first-second"; its connotation indicates "the disease of the first child when the second is expected." It is traditionally associated with the early weaning of babies onto a starchy diet when pregnancies are closely spaced. A child suffering from kwashiorkor fails to gain weight, is peevish, and has a poor appetite. Vomiting and diarrhea are common, and mental and physical development may be impaired. A misleading symptom is the swelling of the body (partly because of the enlargement of the liver) and limbs. Left untreated, children with advanced kwashiorkor die.

Fortunately, this form of malnutrition is rare in Western society. Excessive consump-

Improving Protein Intake from Animal and Plant Sources

Twenty different amino acids are found in animals and plants. Most of them can be made within the human body, but eight essential amino acids (ten in children) can be provided only from food. Animal proteins contain all the essential amino acids, but eating meat every day may not be an economic option and is often not the healthiest option because of the high saturated-fat content of some meats. The alternative is to eat vegetables, but the protein from individual plant foods does not contain all the essential amino acids (soy is the exception; it is the one plant food that provides all the essential amino acids). However, if a "cocktail"

of plant foods is consumed, the deficiency of one can be compensated for by another to meet protein requirements. A diet rich in legumes and grains achieves this requirement, through a mutual effect. Beans and peas lack the essential amino acid methionine, but are good providers of lysine; grains, by contrast, are relatively poor sources of lysine but contain abundant methionine. The only problem with relying on plant foods as the sole protein source is that the amount of plant food that must be consumed can create difficulties for very young children.

Guidelines for Protein Intake

Animal sources (contain all essential amino acids)

- Eat fish very often, or at least twice a week
- Eat lean meat such as skinless turkey breast, skinless chicken breast, fillet steak, or lamb fillet often (poached, boiled, steamed)
- Eat medium-fat meat such as chicken legs, rump steak, braising steak, and lamb cutlets moderately often (grilled, stewed, roasted)
- Avoid or eat only occasionally meat with high fat content, such as sausages, cold cuts, pâté, marbled beef, and bacon
- Eat eggs and low-fat dairy products often, including cheese, yogurt, milk

Plant sources

To ensure adequate essential amino acids, eat:

- Legumes: peas, chickpeas, black-eyed peas, lentils, beans such as soy beans (and soy products including tofu, edamame, and soy milk), kidney beans, pinto beans, broad beans, black beans, lima beans, navy beans, mung beans

With

- Grains: rice, wheat, corn, rye, oats, barley, millet, buckwheat, spelt, quinoa

tion of protein is more likely to be the problem in countries like the United Kingdom and the United States. Proteins can indeed be as fattening as carbohydrates. Excess amounts can be converted into fat or glucose and stored if the protein is not used immediately for energy. Proteins supply 4

calories per gram, the same amount as a gram of carbohydrate. Again, the emphasis should be on moderation in consumption.

Meat, fish, eggs, liver, and kidney are all good sources of protein, as are legumes, or peas and beans. Although meat, fish, and eggs are easily digested, legumes such as beans, peas, and lentils are less so. The lower digestibility of peas and beans makes them less effective as a protein source in areas or countries where the total intake of protein is low because of poverty. This is also a factor to be taken into account in vegetarian diets.

The association of animal protein with animal fat and the advice to reduce the intake of saturated fats have led many people in recent times to avoid meat. However, this does not mean that all meat should be avoided. Red meat provides all the essential amino acids and is also a good source of iron, zinc, and vitamins, especially B-12 and retinol (vitamin A; see the section on vitamins later in the chapter). The solution is to eat meat while avoiding fat. Lean meats include poultry and game. It helps to remove the skin or any visible excess fat before cooking meat. Eating fish at least twice a week reduces consumption of saturated fats while providing important minerals and vitamins. Eating a wide variety of different proteins in moderate proportions is the best way to insure that you have a balanced and complete diet.

How much protein do we need to consume? As with other major constituents of the diet, the recommended intake of protein varies between countries, genders, and age groups. Differing lifestyles can also have a major influence. Generally, suggested daily intakes are set higher than the body's minimum requirement because a very low protein diet carries a risk of vitamin-B and iron deficiencies. One guideline says between 10 and 15 percent of total calories should come from protein. On this basis, for an average woman between ages 25 and 50, who consumes about 2,200 calories per day, the recommended daily protein intake would be between 55 and 83 grams. In the United Kingdom, the recommended daily intake of protein for this age group is 72 grams. In the United States, by contrast, the guideline says to multiply body weight in kilograms by 0.8; the resulting number is the recommended daily intake of protein, in grams. (To determine body weight in kilograms, divide body weight in pounds by 2.2046.) On this basis, for a woman weighing 140 pounds (63.5 kg), the recommended protein intake would be only 51 grams per day.

Present Dietary Patterns

With increased affluence and the availability of convenience foods, the average diet in the West deviates somewhat from the ideal. A U.S. government–sponsored survey of the dietary habits of 16,000 adults shows the following ways in which what Americans eat deviates from recommendations:[12]

- **Grains:** Only about one-half of Americans eat the six to eleven daily servings of grain recommended by the Food Guide Pyramid, and most Americans eat only one serving of whole-grain foods per day.

- **Fruits and vegetables:** Americans eat about three servings of vegetables daily, and one to one and a half servings of fruit. The Food Guide Pyramid recommends three to five servings of vegetables and two to four servings of fruit.

- **Fats:** U.S.-government guidelines recommend that no more than 30 percent of calories come from fat; about two-thirds of Americans eat more fat than this. In addition, U.S.-government guidelines recommend that no more than 10 percent of total calories come from saturated fat; about 60 percent of Americans eat more than this.

- **Sugar:** Americans consume an average of 20 teaspoons of added sugars per day, accounting for 16 percent of calories. (Most experts recommend that no more than 5 to 10 percent of calories come from sugar.)

- **Salt:** U.S. guidelines recommend that sodium intake be limited to 2,400 milligrams (mg) per day. Yet the average intakes for Americans from food alone (i.e., not counting salt added at the table) are over 4,000 mg for men and almost 3,000 mg for women.

- **Body weight:** More than one-half of American adults are overweight, based on a body mass index (BMI) of 25 or more (see Chapter 2 for a discussion of BMI).

- **Physical activity:** Twenty-eight percent of men and 44 percent of women say they rarely or never exercise vigorously.

It has also been shown that the total meat consumption (including poultry and fish) in the United States has grown nearly 14 percent since 1970. In 1999, about 201 pounds were consumed per person a year, or 8.8 oz a day. This was significantly more than the two daily servings (not more than 6 oz) recommended for those with a total daily calorie intake of 2,200 calories or even the three daily servings (not more than 7 oz) recommended for those with a higher recommended daily intake of 2,800 calories.[13]

Dietary patterns in other affluent countries show similar trends. In the United Kingdom, for example, carbohydrates make up around 42 percent of the total calorie intake, fat accounts for 38 percent, protein 15 percent, and alcohol 5 percent.

By contrast, using the WHO's recommendations and assuming a total recommended caloric intake of 2,200 calories per day, the daily diet of an average woman between 25 and 50 years of age should consist of about 300 grams of carbohydrates (55 percent), 37 to 74 grams of fat (15 to 30 percent), and 55 to 83 grams of protein (10 to 15 percent). For a man within the same age group with a total recommended daily intake of 2,900 calories, the diet should consist of about 400 grams of carbohydrate, 48 to 96 grams of fat, and 73 to 109 grams of protein.

Remember that these are estimates derived from population averages. Adjustments need to be made for individuals according to weight, height, lifestyle, and especially levels of physical activity. In fact, the calculation and development of individual diets is probably best left to a dietician. If there is a need to reduce weight, then the total caloric intake should be lowered by reducing the carbohydrate, fat, and protein content of the diet. If more of one food within a particular category is eaten, an adjustment of other foods in the same category would be required to balance the diet. Other variations may stem from cooking methods.

To improve our diets, several points emerge clearly. We need to cut back on the consumption of sweets and desserts, which are the sources in our diets of most of the sugar and fat that is nonessential. Where possible, low-fat products and monounsaturated and polyunsaturated fats should be used in place of saturated fats. Complex carbohydrates should account for the bulk of the food eaten.

The subject of food and diet is not just about weight control; it is also about good health through the consumption of a balanced diet (see the Food Guide Pyramid on page 175.) Rather than count grams and calories, a person should observe the basic principles of healthy eating:

- Avoid eating more than you need to maintain a healthy weight
- Eat a wide variety of foods
- Eat plenty of fruits and vegetables
- Eat plenty of foods rich in complex carbohydrates and fiber
- Avoid foods that contain a lot of fat
- Avoid sugary foods and drinks

Dietary Intake for Sports

The amount and type of food eaten during training, as well as the timing of a precompetition meal, exert a major influence on athletic performance. The energy requirement of athletes depends on the activity. Activities such as bowling and golf consume between 250 to 350 calories per hour, but strenuous ones such as running, soccer, skiing, and swimming burn 350 calories or more per hour. (For any activity, the exertion will vary depending on the indi-

Total Daily Energy Intakes Required for Intensive Training in a Number of Different Competitive Sports

Sport	Average body weight (kg)*	Estimated daily intake (calories)
Bicycle racing	68	5,995
Boxing (middleweight)	63.5	4,675
Cross-country skiing	67.5	6,105
Fencing	73	5,000
Field hockey (men)	75	5,720
Gymnastics	67	5,000
Marathon racing	68	5,940
Pole vaulting	73	4,620
Sailing	74	5,170
Soccer	74	5,885
Sprinting	69	4,675

*To determine body weight in pounds, multiply kilograms by 2.2046.

(Source: *Encyclopedia of Sports Science and Medicine*, American College of Sports Medicine.)

vidual, so the numbers provided here are approximations used to illustrate the differences in energy expenditure between activities.) Total energy requirements of athletes in intensive training are usually significantly higher than for the average person. The total calorie intake for training in competitive sports generally exceeds 4,500 calories per day and can be over 6,000 calories, depending on the number of hours of training and the intensity of the sport.

The intake of carbohydrates for athletes should be at least 60 percent of total calories, increasing for some sports, such as cycling, to 75 percent. Larger amounts of sugar can be consumed because of the need for quick access to glucose. Carbohydrates, which provide this facility, are high in the glycemic index—an indicator of the increase in blood-glucose levels after a food is eaten (see table on page 190). Foods high in the index provide the most glucose. They are favored by athletes because they offer fast replenishment of energy for working muscles, whereas complex carbohydrates must first be broken down to sugars before they can enter the blood for transport to muscles.

Glycemic Index for Selected Foods

Food	Glycemic index
Glucose	100
Cornflakes	80
White rice	72
Potatoes	70
White bread	69
Raisins	64
White spaghetti	50
Oatmeal	49
Peas	47
Whole-grain spaghetti	42
Apples	36
Milk	34
Lentils	29
Soybeans	15

(Source: Hegarty, V. *Nutrition, Food and the Environment.* St. Paul, MN: Eagan Press, 1995; American Council on Exercise, *Group Fitness Instructor's Manual.* Santiago, CA: American Council on Exercise, 2000.)

Generally, foods with a higher glycemic rating are best eaten before the athletic event/exercise, those with a moderate to high rating afterwards, and those with a low to moderate rating even later. It is not advisable, however, to consume sugar *immediately* before an event. This may increase the level of insulin in the blood and hinder the breakdown of glycogen for empowering muscle contractions. During a race, however, especially in endurance sports such as marathon running, sugared drinks can prove advantageous because they help to conserve muscle glycogen.

Carbohydrate loading, or glycogen loading, is a widely used practice when training for endurance sports such as marathons, long-distance swimming, cycling, and cross-country skiing. Eating increased amounts of carbohydrate allows the maximum storage of glycogen in the muscles; athletes usually do so over the final several days before the competition. As the event approaches, training is reduced and often ceases one or two days before. During the reduced-training and rest periods, carbohydrate loading is increased to build up a sufficient store of glycogen in muscles for the event (see table below). Carbohydrate

Carbohydrate Intake During Training for Competition

	Days before event					
	7	6	5	4	3	2–1
Training duration (minutes)	90	40	40	20	20	rest
Calories from carbohydrates (percentage of total calories)	50	50	50	70	70	70

(Source: Adapted from Gatorade Sports Science Institute.)

loading is not suitable, however, for sports such as weight lifting, soccer, and basketball, which rely in large part on explosive releases of energy.

Protein requirements for athletes depend on the sport. In general, more is needed during periods of training, but no agreement appears to have been reached on exactly how much. Until recently, a suggestion of 1 gram per kilogram of body weight was the norm (25 percent more than the 0.8 g/kg body weight recommended by the WHO for an average adult). Now, some experts suggest increasing the recommended protein intake for endurance sports to between 1.2 and 1.4 g/kg of body weight.[14] It is believed that without sufficient consumption of protein a loss of muscle mass can occur. As the supply of glycogen diminishes, after some 1 to 1.5 hours of high-intensity endurance activity, muscle proteins begin to be broken down to release energy.

People engaged in bodybuilding may need even more protein. Strength development requires a greater consumption of amino acids to replenish and increase the contractile muscle proteins, myosin and actin; as much as 1.4 to 1.8 g/kg of body weight may be needed. With improved strength and training, however, less protein may be required because of the body's increased capacity and efficiency in conserving protein.

Protein intake in excess of the suggested amounts is not necessary, and nor, according to the International Olympic Committee, are amino acid supplements. It is more important that the intake of essential amino acids be maintained, as these can only be provided through dietary sources. The consumption of saturated fats should be reduced and substituted by unsaturated ones. Although fat is a high-energy nutrient, it takes longer to digest and is not a quick source of energy.

The general advice given by dietitians for athletes is as follows:

- Eat larger quantities of carbohydrates during training and before competition

- Eat more protein to compensate for the increased breakdown of muscle protein during training, but adjust the levels according to the activity

- Eat less fat

- Drink carbohydrate-rich liquids during long events

- Drink carbohydrate-rich liquids after the event

- Eat a small meal two hours before an event

- Drink plenty of water

Recommended Daily Intake of Macrominerals and Microminerals

Macrominerals	Good sources	Males	Females
Calcium	Milk, cheese, yogurt, sardines, herring, anchovies, soy, watercress	1,000 to 1,300 mg	1,000 to 1,300 mg
Chlorine	Table salt	2,500 mg	2,500 mg
Magnesium	Wheat germ, bran, nuts, legumes, spinach, whole-grain cereals, whole-grain bread, cockles, shrimps, whelks	240 to 420 mg	240 to 320 mg
Phosphorus	Meat, fish, eggs, poultry, cereals, nuts, legumes	700 to 1,250 mg	700 to 1,250 mg
Potassium	Dried fruits, avocados, bananas, instant coffee, tomatoes, potatoes, nuts	3,500 mg	3,500 mg
Sodium	Table salt, processed foods, cured meats, sausages, pickles, breakfast cereals, bread, margarine, crackers, brine-cured olives	1,600 mg	1,600 mg

Microminerals	Good sources	Males	Females
Chromium	Liver, meat, brewer's yeast, seafood	25 to 35 mcg	20 to 25 mcg
Copper	Shellfish, liver, cocoa, wheat germ, yeast, Brazil nuts	700 to 900 mcg	700 to 900 mcg
Fluorine	Fluoridated water, tea	2 to 4 mg	2 to 3 mg
Iodine	Marine fish, shellfish, seaweed, iodized salt	120 to 150 mcg	120 to 150 mcg
Iron	Red meat, organ meat (especially liver and kidneys), fatty fish such as sardines, egg yolks, dark-green leafy vegetables	8 to 11 mg	8 to 18 mg
Manganese	Cereals and whole-grain cereals, nuts	1.9 to 2.3 mg	1.6 to 1.8 mg
Molybdenum	Whole-grain cereals, yeast, liver	34 to 45 mcg	34 to 45 mcg
Selenium	Meat, grains, shellfish, dairy products	40 to 55 mcg	40 to 55 mcg
Sulfur	Animal and vegetable proteins containing the amino acids methionine and cysteine	none set	none set
Zinc	Shellfish, poultry, meat, eggs, dairy products	8 to 11 mg	8 to 9 mg

These numbers represent Dietary Reference Intakes (DRIS). DRIs vary with age and, for women, may increase above the amounts listed here during pregnancy and lactation.

Note: mg = milligram, a thousandth of a gram; mcg = microgram, a millionth of a gram.

(Source: Adapted from the DRI reports, U.S. Food and Nutrition Board, Institute of Medicine, National Academy of Sciences, 1997–2001. Reports may be accessed via www.nap.edu.)

Minerals

About sixteen chemical elements, referred to as *minerals* by nutritionists, are essential to health. Some elements, the macrominerals, are needed in comparatively large amounts compared to the trace elements, or microminerals. A balanced diet should supply all the minerals required.

Knowledge about the effects of deficiencies in these essential minerals often comes from medical conditions that interfere with the body's ability to absorb them or that accelerate their loss. But even in healthy individuals the absorption or loss of essential minerals and other nutrients in food can be influenced by what we eat. The tannin in tea and the phytic acid in wheat bran and brown rice, for example, can hinder the absorption of calcium, iron, and zinc. Vitamin D is needed for the absorption of calcium, and vitamin C helps with the uptake of iron.

Some minerals may be needed in larger amounts at certain times in life. For example, women need more calcium and iron during pregnancy, and the loss of magnesium and other minerals during prolonged treatment with diuretic drugs might require supplementation. However, self-prescribed mineral supplements should be approached with great caution because, taken in excess, some minerals can be harmful.

Macrominerals

The most important macrominerals are calcium, chlorine, magnesium, potassium, phosphorus, and sodium.

Calcium

Calcium is essential for the formation of bones and teeth, the transmission of nerve impulses, the maintenance of muscle function, the stimulation of some hormone secretions, and blood clotting. When the intake of calcium is insufficient (or calcium absorption is low because of a lack of vitamin D or some other reason), the body draws on bones for its supply. Calcium deficiency, therefore, results in a loss of bone mass (osteoporosis), back pain, brittleness of bones, and muscle weakness. For the majority of people, a high-calcium diet is not harmful because surplus calcium is not absorbed in the body.

Milk and dairy products are among the best sources of calcium. Some green vegetables (broccoli, watercress, and kale), bean curd (tofu), and the soft bones of fish such as sardines and anchovies are also good sources. Be careful though: Not all dairy products are rich in calcium. Butter, cream cheese, and heavy cream are poor sources of calcium. In addition, spinach and beet greens contain oxalic acid, which makes most of the calcium contained in them unabsorbable.

For adult Americans, the U.S. Food and Nutrition Board has established a recommended daily intake for calcium of 1,000 milligrams. An additional 300 milligrams is recommended for children between the ages of 9 and 18; pregnant and lactating women have even higher needs. Their recommended total daily intake is set at 2,500 milligrams.

Chlorine

Chlorine is a poisonous gas, but combined with sodium as sodium chloride (salt), it plays a key role in maintaining the balance of fluids in the body. Combined with hydrogen, it produces hydrochloric acid, which is secreted by the stomach lining as a very dilute solution (0.5 percent) in the gastric juices. The resulting slightly acidic environment helps the enzyme pepsin begin the breakdown of protein. It also kills many of the bacteria that are taken in with food.

Chlorine is usually consumed and absorbed by the body as a chloride. Table salt is a major source of chloride. These days chlorine deficiencies rarely occur because of the widespread use of salt in processed foods and as a condiment. Any excess chloride is excreted in the urine and sweat.

Some experts recommend a daily intake of chloride of about 2,500 milligrams, but the U.S. Food and Nutrition Board has not set a recommendation.

Magnesium

Magnesium is an important component of bones. It is essential for muscle contractions, including those of the heart, and the transmission of nerve impulses.

Magnesium is widely available in a large range of foods, including wheat germ, bran, soy, whole-grain cereals, legumes, nuts, dates, and figs. Dietary deficiency in magnesium is rare. It can arise, however, as a result of poor absorption by the body or because of excessive loss of fluids. Malfunctioning kidneys or an excessive consumption of alcohol can bring about these two conditions. Symptoms of magnesium deficiency include depression, weakness, cramps, and, in severe cases, muscle twitching, heart failure, and death. By contrast, excess magnesium is harmless because it is not absorbed.

The recommended daily intake of magnesium is a little over 400 milligrams for men and 300 milligrams for women. Children need less. During pregnancy and lactation, larger dosages of magnesium are required.

Phosphorus

Phosphorus, usually in the form of phosphates, is an important component of the body's cells and is vital for bone and teeth formation. The process of calcification described earlier (see Chapter 3) involves the laying down not only of calcium but also of phosphates. Phosphorus is essential for energy release and forms part of the high-energy phosphate bonds, especially adenosine triphosphate (ATP), essential for muscle contractions. It is also vital for the absorption of other nutrients.

Except for liquor, fats, and sugar, all foods contain some phosphorus, with dairy products, meat, fish, and eggs being the richest sources. Preservatives containing phosphates are also added to most processed foods and soft drinks. As a result, dietary deficiency of phosphorus is rare. How-ever, an excess can occur in the diet, which results in poor absorption of calcium and in the depletion of calcium in bones.

The recommended daily intake of phosphorus for adults is around 700 milligrams. Children need about 1,250 milligrams.

Potassium

Potassium is essential for maintaining body fluids and their electrical balance in the cells. Together with sodium, it maintains muscle and nerve function, regulates blood pressure, and maintains a normal heartbeat. It is required for the formation of glycogen and is also involved in protein synthesis.

Almost all foods contain potassium. Particularly rich sources include dried fruits, avocados, bananas, instant coffee, tomatoes, potatoes, and nuts. Cooking methods can affect the potassium content of food. Boiling reduces it significantly—by as much

as half in the case of vegetables. Baking and frying have no effect.

Dietary deficiency in potassium is rare because of its wide availability in foods. It can occur, however, following chronic diarrhea, sickness, and prolonged treatment with diuretics. Any excess in potassium intake is normally expelled from the body in urine. If the body cannot remove the excess, for example in instances of kidney failure, it can inhibit muscle contraction, including that of the heart. Excessively high levels of potassium result in lethargy, slow heartbeat, weakness, and confusion.

Some nutritional experts recommend a daily intake for potassium of 3,500 milligrams, but the U.S. Food and Nutrition Board has not recommended a level.

Sodium

Sodium works with potassium to maintain the fluid balance in body cells and is vital for the functioning of muscles and nerves. In particular, sodium is important for the absorption of glucose.

A rich source of sodium is table salt (sodium chloride). Dietary deficiency is rare because of the wide availability of salt in processed foods, including cured meats, sausages, pickles, breakfast cereals, bread, margarine, and crackers. Eggs, meat, fish, and milk also contain small quantities of sodium. Excessive intake of sodium results in fluid retention. It is also associated with hypertension. By contrast, a sodium deficiency can bring about cramps, low blood pressure, and dehydration.

Adults need about 1,600 milligrams of sodium daily. Typically the problem is an excess rather than a deficiency; most people consume four to eight grams per day.

Microminerals

Among the microminerals, or trace elements, the most important are copper, iodine, iron, selenium, and zinc. Others include chromium, fluorine, manganese, molybdenum, and sulfur. Most trace elements are constituents of enzymes, the catalysts that are vital to the body's metabolism. Because for the most part such minute quantities of the minerals are involved, I have not indicated minimum daily requirements in the discussions below. The only exception is iron, for which the DRI is significant, although still small compared to the macrominerals.

Copper

Copper is needed for blood and bone formation and is especially important during growth. It also aids the absorption of iron. Copper is part of many of the enzymes needed for the formation of proteins in bone, skin, and blood vessels and for the production of melanin, the pigment in hair and skin.

Rich sources of copper include shellfish, liver, cocoa, wheat germ, yeast, and Brazil nuts. Dietary deficiency of this trace element is rare. As in the case of other trace elements, excess intake of copper is toxic, causing diarrhea. Prolonged excess intake can result in liver damage.

Iodine

Iodine is needed by the thyroid gland to produce the thyroid hormones, which govern the development and function of the brain and nervous system and regulate body heat and energy.

Rich sources of iodine are marine fish, shellfish, seaweed, and iodized table salt. A low level of thyroid hormones can reduce both physical and mental capacity. Although not the only cause, a deficiency in iodine can cause the thyroid gland to enlarge and the neck to swell, a condition known as *goiter*. In extreme cases it may become so large as to interfere with eating and breathing and part of the gland may have to be removed surgically. Generally, when the swelling is caused by a lack of iodine, it will subside once the diet is modified and the deficit corrected. Iodine deficiency is generally rare in the Western world.

Iron

Iron is needed for the production of the respiratory pigments hemoglobin in the blood and myoglobin in the muscles. Iron helps to transform beta-carotene, found in fruits and vegetables such as carrots, papayas, and apricots, into vitamin A. It is also vital for healthy bones, cartilage, gums, and teeth.

Good sources of iron are red meat, organ meats (especially liver and kidneys), fatty fish such as sardines, egg yolks, and all dark-green leafy vegetables such as spinach. However, as mentioned earlier, the phytic acid in green vegetables makes most of their iron content unabsorbable by the body. It is estimated that at least ten times the weight of spinach would have to be eaten to get the same amount of iron as from eating beef. Dietary deficiency in iron results in anemia, with its accompanying symptoms of lethargy, paleness, and breathlessness.

The recommended daily intake of iron is 8 milligrams for an adult male and 18 milligrams for an adult female; this increases to 27 milligrams during pregnancy. Iron has a higher DRI for women because of the loss of blood during menstruation. After menopause the DRI is the same for both sexes.

Selenium

Selenium is an essential mineral for maintaining healthy hair, skin, and eyesight. It is part of an enzyme that acts as an antioxidant, interacting with vitamin E to protect body tissues against free radicals.

Free radicals are unstable and highly reactive chemicals, often containing oxygen, that are natural by-products of the body's metabolism. They increase dramatically when the body is subject to stress (including air pollution), infection, excessive exertion, or damage. If left unchecked by antioxidants, free radicals cause serious damage to cells, particularly the cell membrane, and trigger chain reactions that can interfere with the normal biochemistry of the body. They have been implicated in contributing to a wide range of diseases, including cancer, Alzheimer's disease, atherosclerosis, and arthritis.

Selenium also helps in the normal functioning of the liver and in the production of important hormones. The best sources of selenium are meat and grains. Shellfish and dairy products are also good sources.

Zinc

Zinc is needed for the synthesis of protein and nucleic acids (RNA and DNA), the development of the reproductive system, the functioning of the prostate gland, and the healing of wounds. It is essential to the functioning of the immune system. Zinc is essential to the action of many enzymes as well as insulin, the hormone that regulates the levels of sugar in the blood.

Zinc is found in shellfish, poultry, meat, eggs, and dairy products. Whole-grain cereals and legumes are also good sources, but their phytic acid content inhibits absorption.

Zinc deficiency is comparatively rare and usually associated with eating disorders and malnutrition. It can result in dwarfism, delayed wound repair, night blindness, and, when it occurs in childhood, impaired development of the reproductive organs.

Chromium

Chromium assists the absorption of glucose in cells. This makes it particularly important for those suffering from diabetes because it enhances the action of insulin, the hormone that regulates glucose levels in the body. Chromium is also associated with the control of fat and cholesterol levels in the blood.

Liver, meat, brewer's yeast, and seafood are good sources of this mineral.

Manganese

Manganese is needed for bone formation and the functions of many enzymes, including the production of hormones. Grains, including whole-grain foods, and nuts are good sources. Natural dietary intake of manganese is normally sufficient.

Molybdenum

This mineral is important for the normal functioning of many enzymes. It is vital for enzymes engaged in the release of iron from the body's store, the conversion of fat to energy, and the production of genetic material.

Good sources for this mineral are whole-grain cereals, yeast, and liver. No cases of deficiency are known.

Sulfur

Sulfur occurs in all body cells. The adult human body contains about 120 grams of sulfur. It is a constituent of two B vitamins (thiamin and biotin) as well as the amino acids methionine and cysteine. Good sources of sulfur are animal and plant proteins. No cases of deficiency are known.

Vitamins

Vitamins are organic substances which, though needed in only minute quantities, are essential to our well-being and health. (The term *organic* refers here to the fact that vitamins contain carbon; it does not refer to organically grown foods.) Characteristically, vitamins are not produced in the body, but must be supplied in food. A notable exception is vitamin D, but even in this case, if the body fails to produce enough, as is often the case during childhood growth, it must be supplemented in the diet. Unlike carbohydrate, fat, and protein, vitamins do not provide energy or serve as building blocks of the body. Instead, they help drive the metabolism of the body; in this function they act as either coenzymes, substances essential for enzymes to work, or precursors to them.

The impact of diets deficient in vitamins can be traced throughout history, most notably in skeletons with the deformities and demineralization commonly caused by a lack of vitamin D. The knowledge that some foods gave protection against particular diseases was undoubtedly built into folk remedies. Probably the best-known example of a cure of this nature is the discovery in the eighteenth century that eating limes prevented scurvy, a disease affecting the skin and connective tissues. The expression "scurvy knave" in early English literature gives some clue as to the prevalence of the disease, as does the nickname of "limey" for British sailors, who were among the first to benefit from the remedy.

Despite the knowledge that some foods seemed essential to health, the existence of vitamins was only confirmed in the early twentieth century. The word comes from a contraction of *vital amine* to *vitamine* by the chemist Casimir Funk. He discovered that the husk of unpolished rice contained an amine (thiamin) that had properties against beriberi. (Beriberi affects the nerves and skeletal muscles, resulting in nerve pains and wasting; or it reduces the heart's pumping capacity, leading to blood congestion in the veins and swelling in the legs, and sometimes in the trunk and face, caused by an accumulation of fluid.) It was discovered later that other vitamins do not have the same chemical properties or functions and that many do not even contain amines, but the name, now shortened to *vitamin*, came into general usage.

Thirteen vitamins have now been identified. They fall broadly into two groups: fat-soluble vitamins and water-soluble vitamins. Fat-soluble vitamins are vitamins A, D, E, and K. They are so called because they are associated with fatty foods and oils. These vitamins have a greater storage capacity than water-soluble ones and, because they are not excreted, can build up to toxic levels in the body. The water-soluble vitamins include the B vitamins (of which there are eight different ones) and C. Excess quantities of these, by contrast, are excreted in the urine.

Fat-Soluble Vitamins
Vitamin A

Vitamin A, or retinol, is needed for healthy development of the retina of the eye (it is especially important for good night vision), healthy skin, normal cell development, and the maintenance of mucous membranes in the respiratory, urinary, and digestive tracts.

Fish, particularly fish-liver oils, are rich sources of retinol. Other good sources of vitamin A include animal liver, dairy products, margarine, and eggs. Plants do not contain vitamin A, but they do have one or more of the pigments that can be converted to it within the body. Of these, beta-carotene is a particularly good source, although about six times the weight of beta-carotene is needed to produce an equivalent amount of vitamin A. Beta-carotene is also an antioxidant associated with reduced risks of cancer. Good sources of beta-carotene include dark-green leafy vegetables and roots and fruits that are either red or yellow, such as carrots, red and yellow peppers, winter squash, mangoes, and papayas.

Vitamin A deficiency is rare in the developed world, but still presents a serious problem in developing countries, where over 200 million children are at risk. It can lead to blindness or even death in children. It also hinders growth and lowers resistance to infection. Excessive intake of vitamin A, generally above 150 milligrams, is harmful because it is fat soluble and therefore is not easily broken down by the body. By contrast, excessive consumption of beta-carotene is not dangerous, but it can turn the skin yellow. The skin color returns to normal when the consumption of beta-carotene is reduced.

The recommended daily intake of vitamin A is 900 micrograms for an adult male and 700 for an adult female; this amount increases during pregnancy and lactation. The average Western diet provides more than the recommended daily intake of vitamin A. Five grams of liver or 75 grams of butter, margarine, or spinach, for example, each contains 750 microgram equivalents of vitamin A, which is almost the entire daily requirement for a woman.

Vitamin D

Vitamin D (ergocalciferol and cholecalciferol) has three important functions in the body. It increases the mineral content of bones, aids the absorption of calcium, and helps the kidney to conserve minerals.

Vitamin D can be produced in the skin through exposure to the ultraviolet radiation in sunlight; it is also available in some foods, including margarine, fatty fish, and eggs. Dairy foods, unless fortified, have only small quantities of vitamin D and other foods practically none. The winter sunshine of northern latitudes or the highly polluted skies above industrial centers can reduce the production of vitamin D, but people generally do not have to rely solely on food for their supply of vitamin D. Exceptions include the sick and elderly who cannot venture out and those individuals who are bound by tradition or religion to remain completely covered.

Vitamin D deficiency results in rickets (deformity of the bones, particularly the leg bones and spine) in children and osteomalacia (demineralization and softening of the bones) in adults. Vitamin D deficiency is rare in the developed world; overconsumption causes liver damage as a result of excessive calcium in the blood (hypercalcemia).

Vitamin E

Vitamin E is a collective term for substances, the most important of which is alpha-tocopherol, that act as antioxidants, primar-ily protecting fats from oxidation. Vitamin E is essential for maintaining cell structure, for the production of red blood cells, and for the functioning of some enzymes. It protects the lungs from harm by pollutants, and the red blood corpuscles from damage by poisons in the blood. Vitamin E is believed to lower the risk of disorders connected with free-radical damage, such as some cancers, stroke, heart disease, and atherosclerosis. There is also a possibility that vitamin E may slow down the process of aging by slowing down the destruction of biological membranes.

Vegetable oils and foods that are high in fats, such as nuts and wheat germ, are the richest sources of vitamin E. Meat, eggs, lettuce, and other leafy vegetables are other potentially good sources.

Vitamin E deficiency is rare because of its widespread availability in food. It occurs mainly when disorders of the body prevent absorption of the vitamin. When a deficiency does occur, it results in anemia because of the destruction of red blood cells. Prolonged excessive consumption of the vitamin reduces intestinal absorption of vitamins A, D, and K. It might also cause vomiting, abdominal pains, and diarrhea.

Vitamin K

Vitamin K is essential for the synthesis in the liver of substances needed for blood clotting. It is found in green vegetables such as spinach, broccoli, and cabbage, vegetable oils, meat, cheese, and liver. It is also synthesized by bacteria in the gut.

Vitamin K deficiency is rare and is usually caused by liver disorders that interfere with its absorption from food or by drug treatments that inhibit the growth of the intestinal bacteria that produce the vitamin. The resulting impaired clotting of the blood can lead, for example, to nose bleeds, a failure of wounds to heal, and internal bleeding.

Water-Soluble Vitamins
The B Vitamins

The B vitamins consist of a group of eight different vitamins: B-1 (thiamin), B-2 (riboflavin), B-6 (pyridoxine), B-12 (cyanocobalamin), niacin, folic acid, and biotin, as well as pantothenic acid. Niacin shares with vitamin D the distinction of being capable of synthesis within the body, in this case from tryptophan, an amino acid found in many proteins. Most of the B vitamins act as coenzymes; apart from vitamin B-12, they are all involved in the release of energy. Folic acid, together with B-12, is involved in the synthesis of nucleic acids (DNA and RNA) which carry genetic information. B-12 is

Recommended Daily Intake of Vitamins

Fat-soluble vitamins	Good sources	Males	Females
Vitamin A (retinol)	Liver, dairy products, margarine, eggs, carrots, red and yellow peppers, winter squash, mangoes, papayas	600 to 900 mcg	600 to 700 mcg
Vitamin D	Margarine, fatty fish, eggs, fortified dairy products	5 to 15 mcg	5 to 15 mcg
Vitamin E	Vegetable oils, nuts, meat, grains, wheat germ, egg yolks	11 to 15 mg	11 to 15 mg
Vitamin K	Spinach, broccoli, cabbage, vegetable oils, pork, cheese, liver	60 to 120 mcg	60 to 90 mcg

Water-soluble vitamins	Good sources	Males	Females
Vitamin B-1 (thiamin)	Pork, liver, organ meats, whole-grain bread, wheat germ, bran nuts, legumes	0.9 to 1.2 mg	0.9 to 1.1 mg
Vitamin B-2 (riboflavin)	Brewer's yeast, meat, wheat germ, poultry, fish, eggs	0.9 to 1.3 mg	0.9 to 1.1 mg
Vitamin B-6 (pyridoxine)	Meat, poultry, fish, brewer's yeast, grains, nuts, soybeans	1.0 to 1.7 mg	1.0 to 1.5 mg
Niacin (nicotinic acid)	Meat, poultry, legumes, nuts, potatoes, wheat germ	12 to 16 mg	12 to 14 mg
Pantothenic acid	Meat, vegetables, grains	4 to 5 mg	4 to 5 mg
Biotin	All foods, especially liver, peanuts, egg yolks, brewer's yeast	20 to 30 mcg	20 to 30 mcg
Folic acid	Leafy green vegetables, legumes, wheat germ	300 to 400 mcg	300 to 400 mcg
Vitamin B-12	Virtually all animal protein: meat, poultry, fish, eggs, dairy products	1.8 to 2.4 mcg	1.8 to 2.4 mcg
Vitamin C (ascorbic acid)	Fruits and vegetables, especially citrus fruits, black currants, rose hips, kiwis, strawberries, green peppers	45 to 90 mg	45 to 75 mg

These numbers represent Dietary Reference Intakes (DRIs). DRIs vary with age and, for women, may increase above the amounts listed here during pregnancy and lactation.

Note: mcg = microgram, a millionth of a gram; mg = milligram, a thousandth of a gram.

(Source: Adapted from the DRI reports, U.S. Food and Nutrition Board, Institute of Medicine, National Academy of Sciences, 1997–2001. Reports may be accessed via www.nap.edu.)

also involved in the synthesis of fatty acids in the myelin sheath that surrounds nerve cells. The myelin sheath insulates nerves and enables the rapid transmission of nerve impulses.

All the B vitamins occur in meat, poultry, liver, yeast, and yeast extract. With the exception of B-12, they are also found in vegetables and fruits. Vitamin B-12 occurs only in animal products and microorganisms such as yeast.

A well-balanced diet will generally provide an adequate supply of all the B vitamins. Deficiencies arise usually as a result of drug treatments or medical conditions that interfere with absorption. People who have poor diets—rich in sugar and white-flour products—or who have a high level of alcohol dependency may also suffer from deficiencies in one or more of the vitamins. Because vitamin B-12 is found in animal but not vegetable foods, vegans who do not eat animal foods, including eggs or dairy product, are at particular risk. If they do not eat foods fortified with the vitamin, they may need to take supplements.

I have already mentioned beriberi, a deficiency disease caused by a lack of thiamine. That disease has mostly disappeared from the developed world. Prolonged niacin deficiency can cause pellagra, an ailment that causes diarrhea, skin problems, and dementia. This, too, is rarely seen other than in cases of severe alcohol dependency

or when the vitamin is not properly absorbed. More common are conditions associated with a lack of vitamin B-12 because of an inability to absorb the vitamin or, less frequently, because it is lacking in the diet. Shortages as a result of malabsorption, which may be associated with a lack of folic acid, cause pernicious anemia, while a deficient diet results in megaloblastic anemia. In both instances, the oxygen-carrying capacity of blood is reduced because the bone marrow produces abnormally large and deformed red blood cells. Left untreated, these disorders can prove fatal. B-12 deficiency also damages the nerve tracts in the spinal cord, leading to difficulties in walking and even partial paralysis. In vegans, possible damage to the ner-vous system is hidden because their high consumption of folates, compounds derived from folic acid and found in abundance in green leafy vegetables, legumes, and nuts, arrests the megaloblastic anemia and masks the more obvious symptoms of B-12 deficiency.

With the exception of vitamin B-6 and niacin, there are no known harmful effects from excessive consumption of B vitamins because they are normally excreted in the urine. Excessively high doses of vitamin B-6, often prescribed to relieve premenstrual syndrome, mood swings, and bloatedness, can result in nerve damage, causing the ends of the fingers and toes to lose any sense of feeling. Large doses of niacin over extended periods can cause skin flushes and lead to liver damage.

Vitamin C

Vitamin C, or ascorbic acid, is vital for the formation of collagen, a key protein for healthy skin, bones, and supporting tissues as well as the healing of wounds. Vitamin C increases the absorption of iron, thereby helping to avoid iron-deficiency anemia, strengthens the body's immune system, and helps guard against infection. Vitamin C also assists with the synthesis of serotonin, a substance that influences mood and levels of consciousness, and noradrenaline, a hormone that regulates blood flow.

Relatively large amounts of vitamin C are needed. Vegetables and fruits are the best sources, and citrus fruits are particularly rich in vitamin C. Black currants, guava, kiwi, strawberries, and rose hips are also good sources, as are green peppers, Brussels sprouts, watercress, and dark-green vegetables. Vitamin C is difficult to preserve in foods because it is easily destroyed by oxidation and heat. Long exposure to air after peeling or preparing fresh fruits and vegetables or damage such as wilting will seriously reduce the vitamin C content. Overcooked vegetables contain little or none of the vitamin.

Dietary deficiency of vitamin C is rare, but there is a widespread belief, still a matter of scientific debate, that large doses offer extra protection from viral attack and other dangers. Vitamin C cannot be stored in the body, but large doses are retained until the body cells are saturated. The excess is excreted in the urine. Although not normally considered harmful, regular large doses of more than a gram per day can cause upset stomach, cramps, diarrhea, and even kidney stones in susceptible people.

Water

We cannot exist without water. Some 60 percent of the body weight of an adult consists of it. Water is essential to bodily processes and functions. The interface between the air and our lungs is kept continually moist to allow the exchange of carbon dioxide and water for life-giving oxygen. Digestive juices break down the nutrients required for nourishment. The nutrients are transported around the body in the blood, an aqueous solution. About half the volume of blood consists of blood cells and the remainder is a plasma, of which 95 percent is water. Water helps in the regulation of body temperature. It acts as a protective cushion in roles as varied as serving as a barrier for the joints and supporting the fetus within the amniotic sac.

Life is thought to have originated in or around shallow seas; we carry the badge of our origins to this day. The skin protects the body from dehydration. The transition to the land meant that creatures had to conserve water. Removal of the waste products in urine and feces requires water, but the body retrieves as much of it as possible before they are finally expelled. Even so, water is lost and must be replaced, both directly and through the breakdown of food.

An inadequate intake of water can cause headaches, poor concentration, constipation, poor complexion, and, over a longer period, kidney stones. We require about three liters of water per day. Typically, drinks such as milk, tea, coffee, fruit juices, and plain water provide the bulk of our needs, followed by solid foods such as dairy products, bread, cereals, meat, fish, eggs, fruits, and vegetables. Overall, if eight glasses of water are drunk each day and a wide range of vegetables and fruits are eaten, the daily water requirement will be met. If, however, the level of physical activity is high or the weather hot, more is needed to replace an increased loss through perspiration.

Alcohol

Alcohol is not essential to a healthy diet. It is, however, part of the social lifestyle in many societies, especially in the West. Taken in moderation and alongside food, as in the Mediterranean, alcohol may help reduce the risk of coronary heart diseases in men and women. The problem lies with the definition of *moderation*. According to the WHO, alcohol should not be consumed at all, or at the most should not exceed 4 percent of our total daily calorie intake. Even in the case of the latter, incorporating one or two alcohol-free days each week is advisable to enable the body to detoxify itself.

In the United Kingdom, on average, about 5 percent of the total calorie intake per person is alcohol. In some reports, the figure is as high as 8 percent. To keep individual consumption to a moderate level means limiting oneself to just 1 or 1½ units of alcohol per day and never exceeding a maximum of 21 units per week (3 units per day) for men or 14 units per week (2 units per day) for women. One unit is equivalent to twelve fluid ounces of beer, six fluid ounces of wine, or one and a half ounces of liquor.

Alcoholic drinks consist mainly of empty calories—that is, they tend to have little nutritional content. A small glass of wine contains 85 calories and half a pint of beer 175 calories. Worse is the impact alcohol has on bodily functions. Heavy consumption of alcohol reduces coordination and control, inhibits speech, results in dehydration, and impairs decision-making and response patterns. Taken in excess over time, alcohol enlarges the liver, causes cirrhosis, fibrosis, and scarring, and increases the risk for liver cancer. It increases the risks of cancer in other parts of the alimentary system (mouth, throat, esophagus, and stomach). It can also result in personality changes and dependence.

Poor health and nutritional inadequacies are often associated with excessive alcohol consumption because of its diuretic effect, which results in the depletion of vitamins, especially the water-soluble ones. It also interferes with the body's ability to absorb certain vitamins (vitamin B-6, foliate, and thiamin) and minerals (zinc). Broadly speaking, the consumption of alcohol is incompatible with fitness and health.

In this chapter, we have reviewed the major foods, including minerals and vitamins, as well as water, that are required for the maintenance of a healthy body. By adopting the healthy eating guidelines outlined above and by taking regular exercises using the principles discussed in the earlier chapters, we should be well on our way to a healthy lifestyle. There remains one other issue that confronts us all, namely growing old, and how to do so gracefully and with the least pain. Chapter 13, the final chapter, addresses this issue.

13

Exercise and Eating for People over 50

While aging is inevitable, the symptoms are not necessarily insurmountable. If you take good care of yourself, the process of aging can be much more manageable than you might first think. These days, when it comes to aging, people are less inclined to adopt the fatalistic view of "what will be, will be." They want instead to take charge of their destiny. To do so, however, it is important to understand the physical and functional changes that take place in the body with age, their implications, and any special needs arising from them. I have touched upon some of these points elsewhere, but I want to develop them further here. My over-50s class is among the most satisfying that I teach because of the changes I see in the participants, not just in terms of mobility and body shape, but in the broadening of attitudes in terms of what is possible as one grows older.

Aging is not a disease. But life-long stress and hard work take their toll on the human body. Gradually, muscles and other soft tissues lose their strength. The heart becomes less efficient; as a result, cardiac output is reduced, and with it the amount of oxygen delivered to body cells. The lungs also weaken, adding to the problem. The energy available for activities diminishes. Muscle coordination declines because of a decrease in nerve cells. Lean body mass is reduced, causing the basal metabolic rate to fall. The digestive juices are reduced, and the smooth muscle declines in activity and strength. This, in turn, can interfere with the absorption of nutrients and cause constipation. The kidneys function less efficiently, bones and teeth become demineralized, and eyesight and hearing deteriorate.

For women, aging brings a fundamental change—menopause. This loss of reproductive capacity and the cessation of menstruation, following the "emptying" of the ovaries, results from a decline in the reproductive hormone, estrogen. Symptoms associated with it include hot flashes, tingling sensations in fingers and toes, night sweats, mood swings and depression, a loss of bone mass and threat of osteoporosis, and an increased risk of cardiovascular heart disease. Some women fear they are unattractive and less feminine, a worry caused in part by socio-cultural attitudes to this phase in life.

All this may seem daunting, but good eating habits and exercise can help stem the tide, prolonging an active lifestyle and improving the quality of life in general. Just as important, by offering a positive outlook at a time of profound change, these healthy habits can raise the spirits by providing benefits that we all agree are worth working for.

Aerobics: Keep On Moving!

Muscles are never completely lost; they atrophy mainly because they go unused. In-sufficient exercise reduces the workload on the heart, causing the cardiac muscles, like any muscle in the body, to lose strength. As a result, the cardiac output declines, oxygen uptake falls, and the capacity of the lungs diminishes. But these conditions are not confined to the old; the young are similarly affected if they are sedentary, although the full impact may not come to light until later in a person's life.

You must not regard age, any age, as a barrier to exercise. Reaching 50 years of age, for example, does not mean that you have become old overnight. You have just added another year to your life. You have certainly not raised a barrier to activity or started on the fast track to a life of reminiscence from an armchair. It is vital to remain active. Make exercise part of your daily routine, even if it was not so before. Set aside time every day for brisk walks of not less than thirty minutes. Two or three times a week, attend low-impact aerobic or dance classes for the over-fifties. Take up t'ai chi or aqua aerobics.

Pursuits like these will provide the cardiovascular stimulation vital to the health and strength of heart, lungs, and muscles. Regular attendance at exercise classes and routine daily activity will improve blood circulation and provide a healthy injection of endorphins that keep feelings of depression at bay. With the exception of aqua aerobics, which is not weight bearing, these activities will help maintain bone mass. These benefits are vital for women in the menopausal phase. Classes also offer another positive feature: They bring people in the same age group together, where the sharing of achievements and even problems can become an enriching experience.

In pursuing aerobic exercise, care must be taken to build up to activities, especially if you are new to them. Unless you have regularly jogged before, it would be preferable to walk briskly. Reduce or avoid activities that jar the hips, knees, and ankles, such as jumping or similar bouncy movements. Keep joints mobile with a good warm-up before the activity and a thorough stretch afterward. It is more important to maintain the overall continuity, intensity, and rhythm of the movements using big muscle groups, such as the quadriceps and calves, to achieve an effective cardiovascular workout than it is to carry out vigorous moves.

Strength, Endurance, and Stretching

Maintaining muscle tone and strength requires devoting time specifically to strength-building exercises. Most aerobic classes incorporate some form of strength-building routines, but if you are not attending classes and your aerobic activities consist primarily of, say, walking, then set aside 15 to 20 minutes two or three times a week for strengthening muscles. Alternatively, 10 minutes daily might be a better option. It depends on your lifestyle.

It is important to maintain the strength of all our muscles, but some muscles merit special consideration as you grow older. They include

- the back muscles, specifically the erector spinae and the latissimus dorsi
- the abdominal muscles
- the pelvic floor
- the quadriceps

These muscles are especially important for folks over fifty, because their weakness often gives rise to common problems such as back pain, incontinence, and pain in the knees and pelvis/hip.

Back Problems

The causes of back pain are as diverse as the people you consult. Everyone has a different explanation, ranging from strained ligaments to psychological stress. The treatments offered are just as diverse. One thing is clear: Physical-fitness programs can both reduce back pain and create a sense of well-being. They tackle the problem from both sides—the physical and emotional. Personally, I have little doubt that most back problems can be traced to poor posture and incorrect body alignment.

Long hours spent sitting at a desk or working while looking down create future problems for the body's framework. Other contributing factors which add to pressure on the back are the increased weight and greater girth often associated with age and caused by the reduction in basal metabolic rate and lean body mass. When abdominal muscles are strong, they help support the stress borne by the back. A strong transverse abdominus, for example, acts like a corset to keep the body aligned. When it is weak, the lower back has to support the weight of the body, creating great stress in the lumbar region.

The back has yet another constraint. When we stand, the entire weight of the body bears down on the spinal column, compressing the intervertebral discs that lie between the vertebrae. In the morning, the spinal column is longer and a person is taller than in the evening, because lying down to rest reduces the pressure on the intervertebral discs, allowing them to return to their normal thickness.

As muscles shorten and tighten with age, this problem of compression worsens and can become permanent. The cause of this is osteoporosis. Osteoporosis, or the loss of protein matrix tissue from bone, is a natural part of aging that results in a loss of bone density in the skeleton. The back rounds and the head thrusts forward, giving rise to the stereotypical bent frame of the

elderly. Problems such as these do not arise overnight. They can affect the young as well, but the elderly have inevitably spent considerably more time subject to poor body alignment and gravitational pull than a 20-year-old.

To tackle the problem and provide relief for the spinal column, it is important to improve body posture, strengthen the abdominal muscles, mobilize the back, and stretch the back muscles. The exercises below are designed especially to meet the s___ific problems associated with aging, b__ __y can also be used by younger peop__ __ want to improve abdominal-muscle ____ but wish to have some support f_ back while exercising.

Strengthening Abdominal Mu___

The abdominal exercises suggested h___ volve techniques that, as far as I kn__ not used elsewhere. From experienc__ my classes, these exercises work real__ You might like to use music with the r___ to make it more interesting. Choose ___ with a regular but slow tempo. I h__ peated the sequence for getting into ___ body alignment in each exercise to st___ importance and also for easy referen___ gard it as a blueprint that, once ma___ you should not need to refer to ag__ hope is that eventually you will aut___ cally position your body correctly ___ starting the workout.

Scaling the Wall (Abdominal Muscles)

in front of a wall and place both
t, hip distance apart, flat against it.
ke sure that the knees are aligned
ve the hips and the thighs are verti-
to the floor. You should be comfort-
e in this position.

ce the palms by the side of the
d, ensuring that both shoulders re-
in on the floor. This averts the ten-
cy to attempt to reach forward or
ress the palms down on the floor,
ch would pass the stress to the
ds rather than working the abdomi-
muscles.

e a deep breath and exhale, con-
cting the navel toward the spine; the
er back moves toward the floor, and
lower abdomen deflates and tight-
s, tilting the pubic bone up slightly.

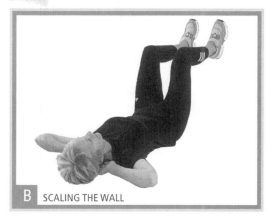

B SCALING THE WALL

The bottom comes slightly off the floor, and the feet push harder against the wall. If this is uncomfortable because the small of the back remains off the floor, place a towel folded flat under this area.

- Hold and then release.

- Repeat the above six to eight times to start with; in subsequent sessions, increase the number of repeats. Vary the contractions; breathe out and contract and then contract again more deeply, breathing out fully in the process, followed by release and then even further release to the original position, breathing in as you do so.

- Exhale to come out of the position, and, if you can, bring your knees toward the chest. Return to even breathing.

- Hold the knees against the chest to stretch out the lower back and release the tension in the abdominal muscles.

These floor exercises might not suit those who suffer from dizziness and/or have difficulties getting down on the floor. If that is the case, perform the exercises standing up: Inhale and exhale, sending the navel toward the spine and allowing the lower abdominal muscles to contract and flatten. Do a "pelvic-floor tilt," tilting the pubis up slightly. Release and return the pelvis to its normal position. Repeat as many times as is comfortable.

The floor version of the exercise can be done without the wall, but using the wall is safer and more effective for those with weaker muscles because it provides support and helps keep the focus on the abdominal muscles. The exercise is also a good starter for those unacquainted with the transverse abdominal muscles. To progress even further, the next stage is to "walk up the wall," contracting the lower abdominal muscles with each step. The technique is not as complicated as it sounds, but it does require practice.

Wall Walk
(Lower Abdominal Muscles)

- Lie in front of a wall and place both feet, hip distance apart, flat against it. Make sure that the knees are aligned above the hips and the thighs are perpendicular to the floor. This time, make sure that the lower leg, from the knee to the foot, is parallel to the floor. You should be comfortable in this position (see photograph accompanying preceding exercise).

- Place the palms by the side of the head, keeping your shoulders on the floor.

- Take a deep breath and exhale, con-

tracting the navel toward the spine; the lower back moves toward the floor and the lower abdomen deflates, tilting the pubic bone up slightly. This is the starting position.

- Breathe in and move your right foot one step up (about 10 inches); then as you place the foot on the wall, exhale, sending the navel toward the back of the spine, and contract the lower abdominal muscles.

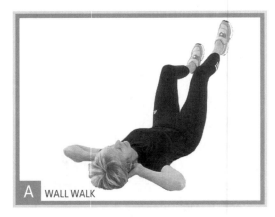

A WALL WALK

- Breathe in and move the left foot a similar distance up the wall; breathe out as you place the foot on the wall.

- Breathe in as you "step down" with the right foot; as you place the foot on the wall, breathe out to contract the lower abdominal muscles.

- Breathe in; step down with the left foot; breathe out.
You have now completed one full set.

- Repeat three additional sets of steps. Increase the number of repetitions in future sessions.

- Exhale and bring the knees to the chest. Hold, stretching out the lower back and releasing the tension in the abdominal muscles.

Pelvic-Floor Exercise

Women can build on the two above positions to strengthen the pelvic floor. When you contract the lower abdominal muscles, focus also on the pelvic floor by tightening the muscles around the vagina, as though you are drawing them inward and upward toward your navel. In the following steps, *the pelvic-floor component is added in italics.*

- Lie in front of a wall and place both feet, hip distance apart, flat against it. Make sure that the knees are aligned above the hips and the thighs are perpendicular to the floor. Ensure that the lower leg, from the knee to the foot, is parallel to the floor.

- Take a deep breath and exhale, contracting the navel toward the spine; the lower back moves toward the floor and the lower abdomen deflates, tilting the pubic bone up.

- *On the next out-breath, contract the muscles around the vagina and the*

sphincter muscle surrounding the bladder neck of the urethra; the bottom comes slightly off the floor and the feet push harder against the wall.

- Release, breathing in.

- Repeat as before.

Men have similar pelvic-floor muscles and can face the same problem of weak bladder control. This occurs, for example, after treatment for an enlarged prostate. They can also benefit from the pelvic-floor exercises described above, with some adjustments, of course, for differences in anatomy. Men should tighten and pull up the muscles of the pelvic floor by imagining they are passing water and then attempting to stop it.

Pelvic-floor exercises should be done daily to avoid problems of incontinence. For those uncomfortable doing the exercise lying down, an alternative is to stand with the feet slightly apart and follow the sequence above, starting with the breathing. (Obviously, the references to the floor would not apply in this variation.) This is equally effective for the pelvic floor, but less so for the abdominal muscles.

Maintaining the Back

The postural muscles in the back are almost continuously contracted in order to hold the body up. These muscles have to be stretched to release the stress exerted on them and to maintain their flexibility. Maintaining the flexibility of these muscles essentially involves retaining their natural length. To keep the back flexible requires more than muscle flexibility; it also requires the "joints"—the junctions between the vertebrae—to be mobile. If they are not mobile, the movement of the spinal column will be severely restricted.

Feline Stretch (Erector Spinae)

 ▪ Kneel, with the knees hip distance apart. Place both palms on the floor, aligning the palms directly below the shoulders, fingers pointed forward. Make sure that the weight of the body is evenly distributed.

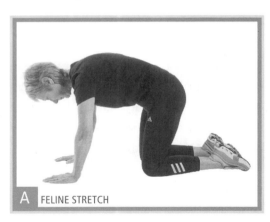

A   FELINE STRETCH

 ▪ Exhale, tucking the chin toward the chest, tucking the base (coccyx) of the spine and the sitting bones under you,

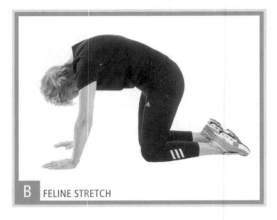

B   FELINE STRETCH

and tucking the tummy in, contracting the navel toward the spine. The body is now curved as though you were an angry cat.

▪ Hold and release, breathing in as you do. You should feel the muscles in your back lengthening from the head to the tail end, opening up spaces between the vertebrae. The trapezius muscles, which lie between the shoulder blades, will also lengthen from shoulder to shoulder.

▪ Repeat three times at least. Each movement should be slow and controlled.

Standing Feline Stretch (Erector Spinae)

For those who have knee problems or find it difficult to kneel, a modified back stretch can be performed standing up.

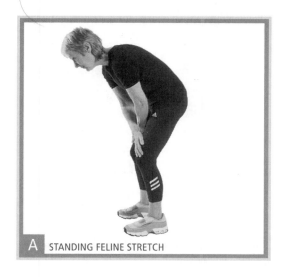

A STANDING FELINE STRETCH

A ▪ Stand with feet hip distance apart; cross your arms and place each hand on the opposite knee or upper thigh.

B ▪ Take a deep breath and exhale. As you exhale, tuck your chin towards your chest, tuck the tail end (coccyx) and sitting bones under, and tuck the

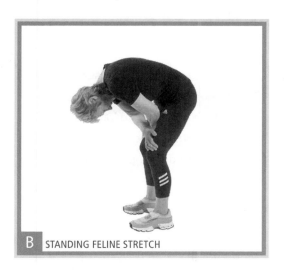

B STANDING FELINE STRETCH

tummy in, sending the navel toward the spine. The body is now curved like an exaggerated question mark.

▪ Hold the stretch, breathing normally, and then release. Return to the normal position, but do not arch your back.

▪ Repeat three times.

Maintaining the Quadriceps

Strong quadriceps help support the knees and assist movements such as climbing steps, walking uphill, sitting down, getting up, especially from a deep armchair, and getting out of cars. The easiest way to strengthen the quadriceps is to climb stairs. However, you might still find it useful to set aside two to three minutes per day to do the following:

Squats with Support (Quadriceps)

▪ Stand with your feet hip distance apart and your body upright, holding on to a support such as the back of a chair or a wall. If using a chair make sure it will not topple over.

▪ Gently bend the knees as though you **B** are going into a sitting position, breathing out as you do so. Bend your legs, if possible, to about 45 degrees, so that the knees in this position are aligned above the toes but not beyond them.

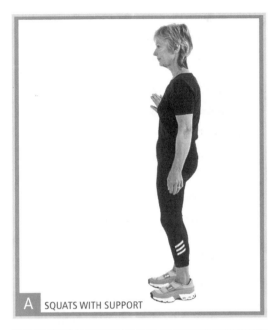

A SQUATS WITH SUPPORT

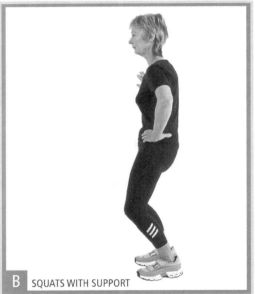

B SQUATS WITH SUPPORT

- Gently return to a standing position. The movements should be slow and controlled. You should feel the upper

part of the thigh, the quadriceps, working.

- Repeat. The number of repetitions depends on the individual. Start with a comfortable six or eight squats and build up to as many as you can sustain. You might try for 12 to 15 a day, but if this is too ambitious, do a set of 6, rest, and do another 6.

The slower the squat, the more difficult it is. When you have mastered the exercise, you can try going down in two stages and coming up in two stages, pausing after each one. If you are strong and have good balance, do the squats without a chair, balancing the body with arms stretched forward.

Thigh Stretch with Support (Quadriceps)

This is an exercise for stretching out the quadriceps after the squats.

- Hold on to a wall or chair for support.

- Keeping the knee of the supporting leg soft, bring the heel of the other leg toward the bottom, grasping the ankle with the hand. Keep the knees together and tilt the pelvis forward to effect a better stretch for the quadriceps.

- Hold and release. Breathe evenly throughout.

- Repeat the stretch on the other side.

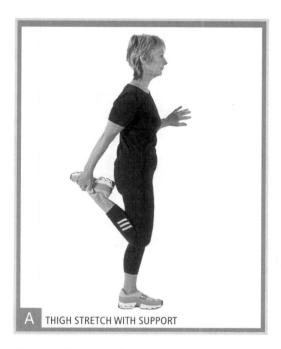

A | THIGH STRETCH WITH SUPPORT

Extras for the Brave

The strengthening and stretching exercises outlined above are geared toward the special needs associated with aging. Many individuals, however, may wish to do more. How much you do will depend on your level of fitness; it is difficult to generalize. The example of Helen Klein in Chapter 4 gives heart to all of us.

I have included in the following exercises the use of a wall. A little support to start with does no harm and can help in maintaining correct body alignment, because by using a wall you can judge if you are standing straight or not. If even these exercises are too easy for you, consider trying the exercises described in Chapters 9

and 10. However, although the following exercises look deceptively easy, if they are executed well, using correct body alignment, they may prove more difficult than you think. For this reason they are also suitable for younger people.

Remember, you can always adjust the intensity of the exercise according to your needs. Now turn on the music!

Back Leg Lift (Gluteals)

- Stand facing a wall with your feet no more than hip distance apart.

- Place both hands on the wall for support.

- Take a deep breath; then, as you exhale, let the navel contract toward the back, tilt the hips slightly forward, and extend the right leg behind you. This setup helps to keep the hips stable and prevents you from lifting the leg too far, causing the small of the back to sag. Keep the supporting leg soft, with a slight bend to the knee.

- Lift and lower the extended right leg in a slow and controlled manner, pausing at the end of the lift to work harder. Breathe out as you lift and in as you lower.

- Repeat six to eight times, or as many times as is comfortable.

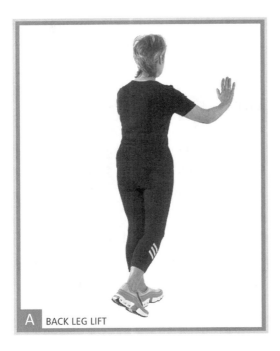

A | BACK LEG LIFT

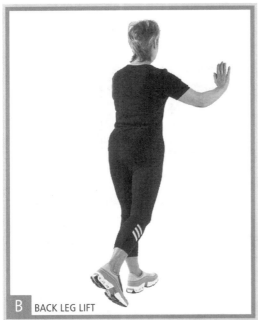

B | BACK LEG LIFT

- Repeat, using the left leg.

You can vary the contraction. If you find that the supporting leg tires easily, then reduce the number of repetitions and perhaps increase the number of sets instead. In this way you will find that there is less stress on the supporting leg. When you become stronger, the stress will eventually disappear.

Leg Curls
(Gluteals and Hamstring)

- Stand facing a wall with your feet no more than hip distance apart.

- Place both hands on the wall for support.

- Take a deep breath; then, as you exhale, let the navel contract toward the back, tilt the hips slightly forward, and extend the right leg behind you. Again, this setup helps to keep the hips stable and prevents you from lifting the leg too far, causing the small of the back to sag. Keep the supporting leg soft, with a slight bend to the knee.

- On the next out-breath, lift the extended leg off the floor, and bend it to bring the heel towards the buttocks. Then straighten it. The movements should be slow and controlled, and the breathing even. Do not apply force

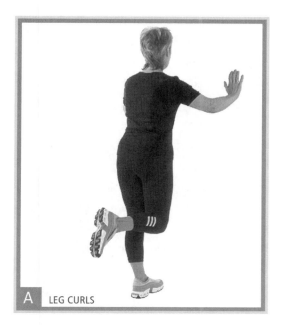

A   LEG CURLS

when bending the leg; for most people the heel will not touch the buttocks.

- Repeat six to eight times, or as many times as is comfortable.

- Change legs.

Side Leg Lift
(Tensor Fascia Latae and Gluteals)

- Stand next to a wall or a strong, firm chair (one that will not topple over), and place one hand on the wall/chair for support.

- Take a deep breath; then, as you exhale, let the navel contract toward the back and tilt the hips slightly forward. This gives the stability you need to

make sure the movement that follows doesn't involve the hip.

- Bring the leg furthest from the wall slightly out to the side, and bend the body slightly towards the extended leg. The knee of the extended leg should be facing forward rather than upward. This is the starting position. By bending toward the leg that you are working, you relieve the supporting leg from carrying the full weight of the body.

- Lift and lower the extended leg in a slow and controlled manner. This "working leg" should be straight, but do not lock the knees of either leg. Breathe out as you lift and in as you lower.

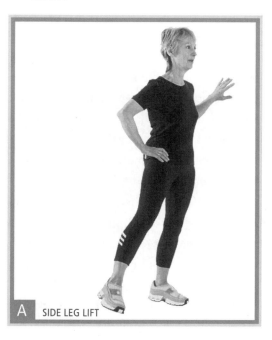

A   SIDE LEG LIFT

- Repeat six to eight times or as many times as is comfortable.

- Change legs.

You should feel a tightening of the buttocks and the outer thigh muscle. Beginners who find that the supporting leg tires easily should reexamine their body alignment. One of the most common problems is keeping the supporting leg rigid and leaning towards the wall/chair. This brings the whole weight of the body onto the supporting leg, resulting in stress. Also remember to keep the supporting leg soft. Another mistake is to lift the working leg using the hip, so do check your body alignment to make sure you're not hiking your hip up as you lift your leg. It may also be necessary to do fewer lifts per set and to incorporate lots of rest in between sets. When you gain strength, you will find that the stress on the supporting leg disappears and all the workout is on the leg desired! Take heart—even those in their early twenties can have difficulties initially getting into the right position.

As you gain strength you can increase the number of repetitions or sets of all these exercises. Vary also the speed in the lifting and lowering of the leg, but take it easy to start with; give top priority to perfecting the technique. Then build up to more reps and sets.

It is important to stretch out the leg muscles after the exercise. In particular, the calves and the hamstrings have to be lengthened to maintain their flexibility. Any of the stretches outlined in Chapter 6, on warm-ups, can be used if you find it difficult to stretch on the floor, but hold them marginally longer than the chapter recommends (12 to 15 seconds), and use support such as a wall or chair if necessary. The main aim in stretching after exercise is to return the muscles to their original length, rather than to develop their length. Since these stretches have been described earlier, I provide only two illustrations in this chapter to show how a wall (or chair) might be used for support in stretching out the calves and hamstring at the end of a workout.

For those who have no difficulties going to the floor and who are supple, some of the floor stretches illustrated in Chapter 10 on flexibility training may be used. However, they are advanced, and I suggest using only the static position for stretching the hamstring, at least to start with (see page 145).

Calf Stretch Using Wall (Gastrocnemius)

- Stand facing a wall, about one foot away (i.e., with enough space to lean forward towards it).

- Lean forward and place both hands on the wall for support.

- Take a deep breath and exhale, tucking in the tummy and placing one leg

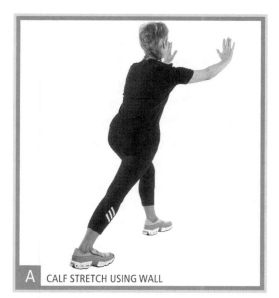

A CALF STRETCH USING WALL

behind you, bending the front leg in the process.

- The knee of the bent leg should be aligned above the ankle to avoid any stress on the knee.

- The heel of the extended leg should be on the floor, with toes pointed forward for proper alignment.

- The upper trunk of the body is inclined slightly forward (a vertical position would stress the lower back).

- Hold the stretch on the calf of the extended leg for 12 to 15 seconds, and release.

- Repeat on the other side.

You will find that, supported by the wall, you can hold the stretch for more than 12

to 15 seconds without discomfort. You can also stretch the calves even more by taking the leg further out behind you.

Hamstring Stretch Using Wall

- Stand with your side to the wall and place one hand on the wall for support.

- Take a deep breath; as you exhale, bend the leg nearest the wall (the supporting leg) and extend the other leg in front. You should be absolutely stable and comfortable.

- Bend the body slightly, placing the free hand on the thigh of the supporting leg for greater stability, and gently lower the upper trunk forward until you feel a stretch in the hamstring of the extended leg. Hold for 12 to 15 seconds

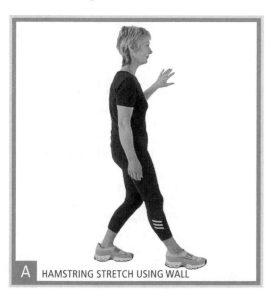

A HAMSTRING STRETCH USING WALL

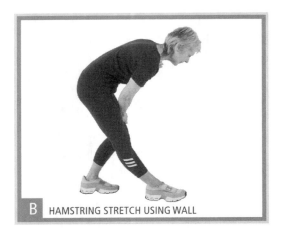

B   HAMSTRING STRETCH USING WALL

and release. Be careful not to "slump" the body when lowering the torso.

- Gently return to the upright position.

- Repeat on the other side.

Appendix 3, Program 5 provides suggestions for structuring exercise programs for folks over 50.

Nutrition for Changing Needs

Nutritional needs change with age. The decline in lean body mass and basal metabolic rate, together with reduced physical activity, mean that the body's energy requirement diminishes. If the same calories are consumed as in earlier years, the result will be increased weight and even obesity. Energy requirements can fall by as much as 5 percent for each decade after 40 years of age (see Chapter 4, page 54, for the recommended daily calorie allowance).

Although an older person's total energy requirement decreases, other nutritional needs increase because of the greater need for regeneration and repair. While the amounts of vitamins and minerals required by those over 50 years of age are about the same as those of a younger adult, the need for protein increases. In the United States, for example, a consumption of 60–75 grams of protein a day, depending on body weight, is recommended by the American Dietetic Association for those over 50. This figure compares with the average recommended daily allowance of 46 grams of protein a day for women and 56 grams a day for men in the United States. It is to be noted that no official recommended daily protein intake has been set for the elderly and different nutrition organizations in the United States have slightly different suggestions on the levels to be consumed. Overall, however, the view appears to be that the elderly would benefit from a daily protein intake that exceeds the 0.8 grams per kilogram of body weight recommended for younger adults. In the United Kingdom no additional quantities of protein are suggested, but the recommendation for the elderly to consume foods that are concentrated sources of proteins, vitamins, and minerals reflects a similar view. This emphasis on the need for a more nutritious diet is seen also in the guidelines on eating habits for the elderly in Japan. They are encour-

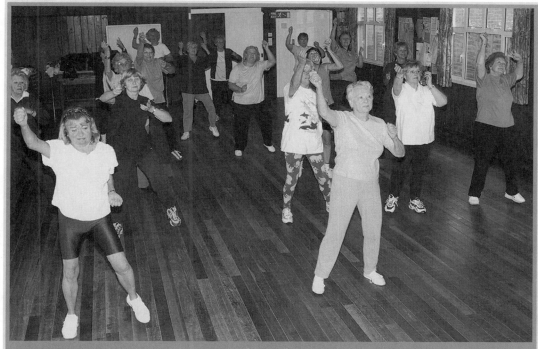

A 50+ Exercise Class in Action
I lead an over-50s class in a local hall. Such classes offer a social occasion as well as an opportunity to improve or maintain fitness and health. Attention to general well-being is an important aspect of fusion fitness.

aged to "eat side dishes first," rather than the main staple, rice, and to "eat every kind of food."

The increased requirement for nutrients combined with a decreased ability of the digestive system to absorb them makes it vital to choose foods of high nutrient density that are easy to absorb. Elderly people have difficulties digesting and absorbing calcium, vitamin B-12, vitamin C, and iron. Older people often develop difficulties digesting milk because the body no longer produces

enough lactase, the enzyme that digests lactose in milk. In some cases the medication taken to combat illnesses associated with aging interfere with the absorption of calcium. Corticosteroids prescribed for rheumatoid arthritis, for example, decrease calcium absorption and increase its excretion in the urine. In the United States, the recommended daily intake of calcium for adults age 51 and older is 1,200 milligrams, compared to the 1,000 milligrams recommended for younger adults. It is important, therefore, to include in the diet foods that are good sources of these nutrients. Eating aged cheeses that are low in lactose, eating yogurt with active cultures, and drinking lactose-reduced milk or buttermilk are some suggestions for those with problems digesting milk.

Replenishing vitamin B-12 is thought to help reverse lapses of memory and improve coordination and balance because of the role it plays in protecting nerve cells. Incorporating a wide range of animal protein in the diet should meet the requirements of both the amino acid lysine and vitamin B-12. Although a balanced diet should provide an adequate supply of vitamin B-12, supplements might be needed by individuals undergoing treatment with antibiotics.

Besides the particular nutrients discussed above, it is also important to ensure a balanced intake of all vitamins and minerals (see tables in Chapter 12). These are as important for the elderly as they are for the young. In the United States, people over 50 are encouraged to boost their consumption of antioxidants. Vitamins C and E are important antioxidants that help mop up the harmful free radicals that can damage body cells and affect health. Supplements are not really needed if an individual eats plenty of fruits and vegetables. A good rule of thumb is to have at least five servings of fruits and vegetables a day. Medical advice should be sought before taking any supplements.

Foods high in sugar should be avoided because they only contribute calories. An easy step is to stop drinking sweetened beverages. The same is true of fatty foods, although essential fatty acids (see Chapter 12) must be eaten because of their roles in hormone production and the nervous system. It is important, therefore, to be selective with fat consumption. The consumption of saturated fats such as hard animal fats should be reduced in favor of unsaturated fats of the kind found in fish oils and in vegetable oils such as sunflower and olive oil. Sodium consumption should be moderated because of its association with hypertension. One effective way is to gradually reduce the salt used in cooking. Saltiness is an acquired taste that can be reversed with time. Salt with reduced sodium is also available.

The weakening of the smooth muscles of the gastrointestinal tract that comes with age often results in constipation. To offset this trend elderly people should ensure that they have sufficient fiber in their diet. Soluble fiber helps lower cholesterol and manage blood glucose levels, while insoluble fiber alleviates digestive disorders and may help prevent colon cancer. Adequate fluid must also be consumed to maintain the water balance of the body and to contribute to regular bowel habits. The requirement to drink at least eight glasses of water a day remains unchanged with age. Unfortunately, many older people do not drink enough because of the discomfort associated with a full bladder and weak bladder control.

The following simple guidelines should prove useful to you by helping you arrive at a suitable diet and a sensible pattern of food consumption.

To help with digestion and the absorption of nutrients:

- Eat regularly and often

- Do not miss meals

- Eat small quantities at each meal

- Eat and chew slowly

To avoid constipation and improve the efficiency of the kidneys and gastrointestinal tract:

- Drink plenty of water, but in small quantities. The excess gas in the digestive system that causes feelings of discomfort and bloatedness is frequently a result of swallowing air when eating and drinking

- Moderate the consumption of tea and coffee

- Reduce the intake of refined carbohydrates such as sugar

- Incorporate lots of fiber in the diet

Some Beneficial Foods for Seniors*	
Bean sprouts	Economical, good source of vitamins C (a single helping provides ¾ of adult RDA) and B complex, easily digestible protein, produces less intestinal gas than unsprouted beans, low in calories
Chicken	Economical, low in fat, easily digestible protein, rich in vitamin B (without skin)
Dried fruits	Good source of fiber, vitamin A, iron, calcium, and energy
Fish, especially oily	Excellent source of vitamins A and D, omega-3 fatty acids, protein, iron (sardines, mackerel, salmon)
Beans, peas, and lentils	Eaten with grains, these provide a good source of easily digestible protein, B vitamins, and fiber
Strawberries	Soft and easily eaten, rich in vitamin C and beta-carotene, help to encourage the excretion of uric acid associated with gout and arthritis
Garlic	Lowers cholesterol, reduces blood pressure, protects the heart, helps fight infections, and is believed to neutralize cancer-causing chemicals
Turnips	Eliminate uric acid

* This is not a complete or exhaustive list. It highlights just a few selected foods that meet the requirements and problems generally associated with aging.

- Avoid excess consumption of salt
- Moderate the consumption of alcohol

To avoid unnecessary weight gain:

- Avoid foods and drinks high in sugar
- Avoid foods high in saturated fat

To ensure adequate nutrition intake:

- Eat small quantities of a wide variety of foods
- Include in the daily diet:
  - carbohydrates and starches, especially whole-grain products
  - lean meat, poultry, fish (especially oily fish), or eggs
  - dairy products
  - vegetables and fruits
  - peas and beans

To ensure that the nutrients in foods can be absorbed, special attention needs to be paid to food preparation. Soups, for example, are a good medium, because they are easy to consume and digest and they also provide fluid. Mincing lean meat or poultry is ideal for those who experience problems chewing. Steaming and grilling reduces the need for added cooking fat, and the high temperatures help seal in the nutritional goodness of the food.

Some people prepare food with a scale for weighing portions and a list of caloric contents, but there is really no need to do so. With experience and a little common sense it will soon be easy to strike a happy balance in your daily diet. Do not be afraid to experiment with new dishes that offer or increase the variety in your diet. Above all else, enjoy your food!

APPENDIX 1

Calculating Basal Metabolic Rate (BMR)

The simplest way to calculate BMR is to multiply 0.9 (women) or 1.0 (men) by body weight in kilograms (to calculate body weight in kilograms, divide body weight in pounds by 2.2046), and then multiply again by 24, the total number of hours in a day. This was the formula used as an example in Chapter 4. The lower factor used for women is based on the fact that their energy expenditure is generally smaller than that of men because of differences in body composition.

In the example given in Chapter 4 of a woman weighing 63 kg, the estimated BMR is:

$63 \times 0.9 \times 24 = 1{,}361$ calories

More elaborate formulas exist for the calculation of BMR. The Harris-Benedict Equation, based on a biometric study of basal metabolism in the United States, takes into account sex, age, weight, and height as follows:

Males $66 + (13.7 \times W) + (5 \times H) - (6.8 \times A)$

Females $655 + (9.6 \times W) + (1.9 \times H) - (4.7 \times A)$

where W = body weight in kilograms (to calculate body weight in kilograms, divide body weight in pounds by 2.2046)

H = height in centimeters (to calculate height in centimeters, multiply height in inches by 2.564)

A = age in years

Thus, a 40-year-old woman weighing 63 kg and 163 cm tall (about 5' 4") has an estimated BMR of:

$655 + (9.6 \times 63) + (1.9 \times 163) - (4.7 \times 40) = 1{,}382$ calories

Perceived Rates of Exertion	
Age group (years)	Formula for BMR
Males	
10–17	17.7 W + 657
18–29	15.1 W + 692
30–59	11.5 W + 873
Females	
10–17	13.4 W + 692
18–29	14.8 W + 487
30–59	8.3 W + 846
where W = body weight in kilograms	

In the United Kingdom, BMR calculations applied by the Department of Environment, Food, and Rural Affairs (DEFRA, previously MAFF) take into account sex, age group, and weight, using the following formulas:

Using the same example of a 40-year-old woman weighing 63 kg, the estimated BMR is:

$(8.3 \times 63) + 846 = 1{,}369$ calories

As you can see, differences in BMR occur according to which formula is used to make the calculation.

APPENDIX 2

Calories and Joules: An Explanation

This book uses the calorie as a measure of food energy rather than the international standard unit, the joule, because of the widespread use of the calorie in the food industry and in popular literature related to food and diet. The joule was adopted as a measure of energy because the value of the calorie varies slightly according to the temperature of the water at which measurements are made. For ease of calculation, however, one calorie (that is, one "true" calorie or "small" calorie; see explanation in next paragraph) is taken as being equivalent to 4.19 joules.

To add to the confusion, when popular literature uses the term *calorie*, what is really meant is *kilocalorie* (kcal), which equals 1,000 "true" or "small" calories. This is because the true calorie is a relatively small unit of measure. In some books, the term *Calorie*, with a capital letter, is used to denote the kilocalorie. However, in line with most popular literature on food and nutrition published in the United States, this edition of *Fusion Fitness* has adopted the convention of referring to the kcal as *calorie*—with no capital letter.

What does all this mean in terms of your everyday life? It means that the cookie you're eating actually contains 150,000 calories! (But only 150 Calories—or what this book simply calls calories.)

Training Programs

How you structure your own training program depends on what you seek from exercise. Numerous variations and combinations can be made of the different exercises described and illustrated in the book. The following are only suggestions; you may wish to modify the combination as well as the number of sets or reps of the different exercises you perform. A suggestion of 1 x 8 means 1 set of 8 reps; sometimes a range of reps, for example 8–10, is suggested. You should listen to your own body to know what is right for you.

The exercises are structured to provide training to all the major muscle groups, targeting common problem areas. They are sequenced in a way that minimizes the need to change position. For example, there are instances when it is more convenient to perform different exercises on different muscle groups of both legs while lying on the same side before changing positions.

You will need a mat—preferably nonslip—for the floor exercises.

Program 1 (1 hour)

All-around fitness—cardiovascular improvement, motor skill, muscle strength, and endurance and flexibility training

This program is divided three components consisting of a warm-up/aerobic section (25 minutes), toning (25 minutes), and stretching/relaxation (10 minutes).

1. Warm-Up/Aerobic Training (Lively, Motivating Music)

If you are doing this on your own and at home, you might find it easier to combine the warm-up with the aerobic training. Start with, say, a gentle/brisk march to music, and progress to a gentle dance, adapting the various moves such as side steps, heel digs, grapevine, and box step to a simple routine. One simple method is to choose dance steps that add up to counts of eight. A rumba, mambo, or foxtrot are examples. Repeat the moves until you feel warm and pliable.

Alternatively, you could go for a walk; start out slowly to raise your pulse gradually, and after about 5 minutes increase the speed of the walk until you are walking briskly. Continue for an additional 10 minutes or so, and then head home, still keeping up a brisk pace. Slow down as you approach home.

The very fit individual might wish to warm up with a brisk walk for 5 minutes and a slow jog for 15 minutes, before slowing down again to a walk. Others might find it easier to alternate between a brisk walk and a slow jog every one to two minutes.

At the end of the aerobic activity, do the following:

- static (standing still) mobilizing moves, i.e., rotate hips, circle shoulders, bend sideways, turn the upper trunk, bend the knees, flex and point the feet (see page 71).

- mobilize the neck, i.e., turn the head from side to side in a slow and controlled manner, then bend the head forward and, supporting the back of the head with your palms, gently tilt the head backward to stretch the front of the neck.

- short stretches to prepare (see pages 72–73).

2. Toning: Beginners (Slow Music with Strong Beat)

Exercise	Reps/Duration	Where Described
Squats	1 x 8–10	pp. 124–125
Triceps extension on the floor	1 x 8	pp. 137–138
Chest press or Box push-ups	1 x 10–12 1 x 6	pp. 134 pp. 132–133
Back leg lift	12–16 each side	pp. 115–116
Hamstring leg curl	12–16 each side	pp. 130–131
Inner thigh seesaw	12–16 each side	pp. 122–124
Transverse abdominal squeeze, incorporating pelvic-floor component	1 x 8, rest and repeat	pp. 105–106
Conventional crunch with fusion modification	1 x 8	pp. 103–104
Shoulder to knee	1 x 8 each side	pp. 111–112

3. Stretching/Relaxation

Exercise	Reps/Duration	Where Described
The yawn	8–10 sec.	pp. 151–152
"Z" stretch	10–12 sec.	p. 152
Hamstring	30 sec. each side	pp. 145–146
Thigh and shin-muscle stretch	30 sec. each side	pp. 157–158
Feline stretch	1 x 15 sec.	pp. 148–149
Groin stretch	30 sec.	p. 156
The roll-back (pectoralis)	8–10 sec.	p. 153
The roll-forward (trapezius and latissimus dorsi)	8–10 sec.	pp. 153–154
Relaxation/quiet breathing	At least 2–3 mins.	
The time shown indicates the length of hold		

Program 2 (1 hour)

Strength and Endurance (Toning) Training

This is for intermediate to fairly advanced participants. Also divided into three components, it incorporates a short warm-up (10 minutes), 40 minutes of toning, and 10 minutes of stretch and relaxation.

1. Warm-Up (Lively, Motivating Music)

Brisk march, brisk knee bends, side steps; repeat until you feel warm. Then perform:

- static (standing still) mobilizing moves, i.e., rotate hips, circle shoulders, bend sideways, turn the upper trunk, bend the knees, and flex the feet (see page 71).

- mobilize the neck, i.e., turn the head from side to side in a slow and con-trolled manner; then bend the head forward and, supporting the back of the head with your palms, gently tilt the head backward to stretch the front of the neck.

- short stretches to prepare (see pages 72–73).

2. Toning: Intermediate–Advanced (Slow Music with Strong Beat)

Exercise	Reps/Duration	Where Described
Back arm lifts	1 x 8	p. 139
Scissoring the arms	1 x 8	p. 140
Repeat both exercises		
Pedal and stride resting on elbows	2 x 8 single lifts, up for one	pp. 126–127
	and down for one 1 x 8 double lifts, up for two and down for two	
Change sides and repeat		
Modified buttock lift, feet apart	1 x 8 single lifts + 1 x 8 double lifts + 1 x 8 small pulsing single lifts	pp. 120–121
Modified buttock lift, knees in and out	1 x 8 single lifts + 1 x 8 double lifts	pp. 121–122
Modified buttock lift, knees and feet together	1 x 8 single lifts + 1 x 4 double lifts + 1 x 8 small pulsing single lifts	p. 122
Inner thigh seesaw	1 x 8 single lifts + 1 x 8 double lifts + 1 x 8 small pulsing single lifts	pp. 122–123
Toning the inner thigh, adding the oblique crunch	1 x 8 single lifts + 1 x 8 double lifts	p. 123
Change sides and repeat the two inner thigh exercises		
Floor push-ups half extension	10 singles + 6 doubles (optional)	p. 133
Conventional crunch with the fusion modification	1 x 8 single lifts + 1 x 8 double lifts + 1 x 8 small pulsing lifts	pp. 103–104
Transverse abdominal squeeze, incorporating pelvic-floor component	1 x 12	pp. 105–106
Reverse abdominal squeeze, incorporating pelvic-floor component	1 x 8 singles + 1 x 8 doubles + 1 x 8 small pulsing movements	p. 107
Reverse abdominal squeeze, legs straight	1 x 8 singles + 1 x 8 doubles + 1 x 8 small pulsing movements	p. 108
Side reach	1 x 8 singles + 1 x 8 doubles + 1 x 8 small pulsing movements	pp. 110–111
Back extension	1 x 10	p. 114

3. Stretching/Relaxation

Exercise	Reps/Duration	Where Described
The yawn	8–10 sec.	pp. 151–152
"Z" stretch	10–12 sec.	p. 152
Thigh and shin-muscle stretch	30 sec. each side	pp. 157–158
Feline stretch	1 x 15 sec.	pp. 148–149
Forward bend hamstring and calf	30 sec.	pp. 158–159
Full wide-angle stretch	30 sec.	pp. 160–161
Prayer position	1 x 15 sec.	p. 149
The roll-back (pectoralis)	8–10 sec.	p. 153
The roll-forward (trapezius and latissimus dorsi)	8–10 sec.	pp. 153–154
Relaxation/quiet breathing	At least 2–3 mins.	

The time shown indicates the length of hold

Program 3 (1 hour)

Advanced Strength and Endurance (Toning) Training

This is geared towards advanced participants with strong abdominal muscles. Its three components consist of a short warm-up (10 minutes), 40 minutes of toning, and 10 minutes of stretch and relaxation.

1. Warm-Up (Lively, Motivating Music)

Brisk march, brisk knee bends, side steps; repeat the sequence until you feel warm. Then perform:

- static (standing still) mobilizing moves, i.e., rotate hips, circle shoulders, bend sideways, turn the upper trunk, bend the knees, and flex the feet (see page 71).

- mobilize the neck, i.e., turn the head from side to side in a slow and controlled manner; then bend the head forward and, supporting the back of the head with your palms, gently tilt the head backward to stretch the front of the neck.

- short stretches to prepare (see pages 72–73).

2. Toning: Advanced (Slow Music with Strong Beat)

Exercise	Reps/Duration	Where Described
The barre	1 x 8, pause and repeat, 1 x 8 Change sides	pp. 128–129
or		
Pedal and stride, resting on elbows	1 x 8 single lifts, up for one and down for one 1 x 4 double lifts, up for two and down for two	pp. 126–127
Pedal and stride, full sitting position	1 x 8 single lifts, up for one and down for one 1 x 8 double lifts, up for two and down for two	pp. 126–127

The following five exercises should be done in sequence, first on one side and then on the other side:

Exercise	Reps/Duration	Where Described
Straight-back leg extension	1 x 8 single lifts + 1 x 8 double lifts + 1 x 8 small pulsing single lifts	pp. 118–119
Right-angle lift	1 x 8 single lifts + 1 x 8 double lifts + 1 x 8 small pulsing single lifts	pp. 119–120
Acute angle moving in	1 x 8 single lifts + 1 x 8 double lifts + 1 x 8 pulsing single lifts	p. 120
Inner thigh seesaw	1 x 8 single lifts + 1 x 8 double lifts + 1 x 8 small pulsing single lifts	pp. 122–123
Toning the inner thigh, adding the oblique crunch	1 x 8 single lifts + 1 x 8 double lifts	p. 123

After completing the sequence on both sides, continue with the following:

Exercise	Reps/Duration	Where Described
Floor push-ups, half extension or full extension	1 x 10 singles + 1 x 6 doubles	pp. 132–133
Transverse abdominal squeeze, incorporating pelvic-floor component	1 x 12	pp. 105–106
Reverse abdominal squeeze, incorporating pelvic-floor component	1 x 8 singles + 1 x 8 doubles + 1 x 8 small pulsing movements	p. 107
Reverse abdominal squeeze, legs straight	1 x 8 singles + 1 x 8 doubles + 1 x 8 small pulsing movements	p. 108
Moon walk I	2 x 8 singles	p. 109
Moon walk II	2 x 8 singles	pp. 109–110
"Z" position	2 x 8 singles	pp. 112–113
Back extension	1 x 12	p. 114
Triceps extension, buttocks off the floor	2 x 8 singles	pp. 138–139

3. Stretching/Relaxation

Exercise	Reps/Duration	Where Described
The yawn	8–10 sec.	pp. 151–152
"Z" stretch	10–12 sec.	p. 152
Thigh and shin-muscle stretch	30 sec. each side	pp. 157–158
Feline stretch	1 x 15 sec.	pp. 148–149
Prayer position	1 x 15 sec.	p. 149
Forward bend hamstring and calf	30 sec.	pp.158–159
Full wide-angle stretch	30 sec.	pp. 160–161
Prayer position	1 x 15 sec.	p. 149
The roll-back (pectoralis)	8–10 sec.	p. 153
The roll-forward (trapezius and latissimus dorsi)	8–10 sec.	pp. 153–154
Relaxation/quiet breathing	At least 2–3 mins.	
The time shown indicates the length of hold		

Program 4 (1 hour)

Stretch and Tone: Intermediate

This is for participants who are familiar with the static stretch positions and are seeking greater strength and flexibility. Its three components consist of a short warm-up (5 minutes), 30 minutes of toning, and 25 minutes of stretch and relaxation. The stretch exercises are organized in a way that allows you to proceed easily from one position to another in a sequence of smooth, flowing movements.

1. Warm-Up (Lively, Motivating Music)

Brisk march, brisk knee bends, side steps; repeat the sequence until you feel warm. Then perform:

- static (standing still) mobilizing moves, i.e., rotate hips, circle shoulders, bend sideways, turn the upper trunk, bend the knees, and flex the feet (see page 71).

- mobilize the neck, i.e., turn the head from side to side in a slow and con-

trolled manner; then bend the head forward and, supporting the head with your palms, gently tilt the head backward to stretch the front of the neck.

- short stretches to prepare (see pages 72–73).

2. Toning (Slow Music with Strong Beat)

Exercise	Reps/Duration	Where Described
Squats	1 x 8 singles + 1 x 8 doubles + 1 x 8 pulsing movements	pp. 124–125
Back arm lifts	1 x 8	p. 139
Scissoring the arms	1 x 8	p. 140
Repeat arm exercises		
The chest press	1 x 10–12	p. 134
Pedal and stride, resting on elbows	1 x 8 single lifts—up for one and down for one; 1 x 4 double lifts—up for two and down for two	pp. 126–127

The following five exercises should be done in sequence first on one side and then on the other side:

Exercise	Reps/Duration	Where Described
Straight-back leg extension	1 x 8 single lifts + 1 x 8 double lifts + 1 x 8 small pulsing single lifts	pp. 118–119
Right-angle lift	1 x 8 single lifts + 1 x 8 double lifts + 1 x 8 small pulsing single lifts	pp. 119–120
Acute angle moving in	1 x 8 single lifts + 1 x 8 double lifts + 1 x 8 small pulsing single lifts	p. 120
Inner thigh seesaw	1 x 8 single lifts + 1 x 8 double lifts + 1 x 8 small pulsing single lifts	pp. 122–123
Toning the inner thigh, adding the oblique crunch	1 x 8 single lifts + 1 x 8 double lifts	p. 123

After completing the sequence on both sides, continue with:

Exercise	Reps/Duration	Where Described
Transverse abdominal squeeze, incorporating pelvic-floor component	1 x 12	pp. 105–106
Reverse abdominal squeeze, incorporating pelvic-floor component	1 x 8 singles lifts + 1 x 8 double lifts + 1 x 8 small pulsing lifts	p. 107
Reverse abdominal squeeze, legs straight	1 x 8 single lifts + 1 x 8 double lifts + 1 x 8 small pulsing movements	p. 108
Moon walk I	2 x 8 singles	p. 109
Side reach	1 x 8 singles + 1 x 8 doubles	pp. 110–111

3. Stretching/Relaxation (Calm Quiet Music)

Lie on your back:

Exercise	Reps/Duration	Where Described
The yawn	8–10 sec.	pp. 151–152
"Z" stretch	10–12 sec.	p. 152
Static and active hamstring stretches	25–30 sec., release and repeat on the same leg. Stretch each side	pp. 145–146
Buttocks stretch	15–20 sec., repeat on other side	pp. 154–155

Between each of the above stretches, bring both knees to the chest, exhaling as you do so, and rock gently from side to side to release the stretches. Breathe evenly as you rock.

Turn over to lie on your front.

Exercise	Reps/Duration	Where Described
Thigh and shin-muscle stretch	30 sec. each side	pp. 157–158
Feline stretch	15 sec.	pp. 148–149
Prayer position	15 sec.	p. 149
Half serpent	15 sec.	pp. 149–150

Repeat the feline stretch, prayer, and half serpent, three times in a smooth fluid manner.

Then, if you wish, go into:

Exercise	Reps/Duration	Where Described
Full serpent	15 sec. + 15 sec.	pp. 150–151
Prayer position	15 sec.	p. 149

Sit up tall, and do the following exercecises:

Exercise	Reps/Duration	Where Described
Wide-angle stretch	20 sec., release and repeat for 30 sec.	pp. 160–161
Stretching in flight	30 sec., release and repeat.	p. 161 Change legs
The roll-back (pectoralis)	10–12 sec.	p. 153
The roll-forward (trapezius and latissimus dorsi)	10–12 sec.	pp. 153–154
Forearm twist	12–15 sec., release and repeat	p. 154
Relaxation	5–7 min.	

Program 5 (20 minutes)

Age 50-Plus Gentle Toning and Stretching

This is for beginners. For those who are used to exercise and have stronger muscles, the following exercise program is still recommended, although support might not be necessary in some of the positions indicated. You should listen to your body. The exercises focus on strengthening and maintaining the flexibility of those major muscle groups that generally pose the most problems as you get older. The duration of the program is just 20 minutes, but I suggest following it at least three times a week, combined with a heart/lung activity, such as walking, swimming, or dancing. If you do the program immediately on returning from a walk, the effect is optimized. If you do not, then you should start with a short warm-up.

Warm-Up (Slow Music with Strong Beat)

Start with a march, followed by side steps and box steps. Repeat the sequence until you feel quite warm. Then mobilize the neck (turn from side to side, tilt from side to side), circle the shoulders, turn the torso, first to one side and then the other, rotate the hips, bend and straighten the knees gently, and flex and point the feet, taking each one in turn. See page 71.

Tone and Stretch (Slow Music with a Good Beat or Light Soothing Music)

Exercise	Reps/Duration	Where Described
Squats with support	1 x 6, rest, 1 x 6. More advanced students should squat without support and increase reps slightly	pp. 215–216
Thigh stretch with support	Hold for 10–12 sec., change legs and repeat	pp. 216–217
Back leg lift	1 x 6, rest, 1 x 6. More advanced students should increase reps (2 x 8) without rest in between	pp. 217–218
Leg curls	1 x 6, rest, 1 x 6. More advanced students should increase reps (2 x 8) without rest in between	pp. 218–219
Side leg lift	1 x 6, rest, 1 x 6. More advanced students should increase reps (2 x 8) without rest in between	pp. 219–220
Hamstring stretch using wall	10–12 sec., release. Repeat for 20 sec. Change legs and repeat	pp. 221–222
Calf stretch using wall	10–12 sec., release. Repeat for 20 sec. Change legs and repeat	pp. 220–221
Standing feline stretch	10–12 sec. x 3	pp. 214–215

On the floor:

Exercise	Reps/Duration	Where Described
Scaling the wall, incorporating pelvic-floor component	1 x 6, rest, 1 x 6	pp. 211–212
Wall walk	2 x 4, rest, 2 x 4	pp. 212–213

To end the session:

Stand with your feet hip distance apart, making sure that the body is aligned and balanced. Inhale, and as you exhale, slowly turn the torso to the right, hold for 6 seconds, then come back to the center. Repeat on left side. Bring both arms above the head and stretch up to the ceiling. Then go into another standing feline stretch, release, and repeat (see pages 214–215). Gently unfold and straighten the body, roll the shoulders, turn the head from side to side, using gentle, even breathing.

Notes

1. Newsholme, E., Leech, T., Duester, G. *Keep On Running*, Chichester, UK: John Wiley & Sons, Inc., 1994.

2. Health Education Authority, UK Sports Council. *Allied Dunbar National Fitness Survey*. London: Belmont Press, 1992.

3. Website sponsored by the American Heart Association: www.justmove.org/fitnessnews.

4. Peeke, P. "When Stress Makes You Fat," *Fitpro*, Aug./Sept. 2000.

5. Stroud, M. *Survival of the Fittest: Understanding Health and Peak Physical Performance*. London: Random House, 1998.

6. Fair, J.D. "Isometrics or Steroids? Exploring New Frontiers of Strength in the Early 1960s." *Journal of Sports History*. Spring 1993, 20(I): 1–24.

7. See also Egger, G., Champion, N., Bolton, A. *The Fitness Leader's Handbook*, 3rd ed. Kenthurst, Australia: Kangaroo Press, 1997; Rosser, M. *Body Fitness: Basic Theory and Practice for Therapists*. London: Hodder and Stoughton, 1999; Donovan, G., McNamara, J., Gignoli, P. *Exercise Danger*. Floreat Park, Western Australia: Wellness Australia, 1988.

8. Stewart, M. *Yoga*. London: Headway Lifeguides, 1998.

9. Hewett, J. *Yoga*. London: Hodder Headline, 1990.

10. Hicks, A., McGill, S., Hughson, R. "Tissue Oxygenation by Near-Infrared Spectroscopy and Muscle Blood Flow During Isometric Contractions of the Forearm," *Canadian Journal of Applied Physiology*, 1999, 24(3).

11. *Trim the Fat from Your Diet*. London: British Heart Foundation, 2000.

12. "U.S. Diets and the Dietary Guidelines 2000," from the website of the U.S. Department of Agriculture: www.barc.usda.gov/bhnrc/foodsurvey/2000dga.html.

13. Accessed from www.nutrition.gov, a portal to nutrition information across the agencies of the U.S. Federal Government

14. Bean, A. "Protein the Powerhouse," *Fitpro*, Feb./March 2001.

Bibliography

Aaberg, Everett. "Full Range Movement, Fact or Fallacy." *Fitpro*, Oct./Nov. 2000.

American Council on Exercise. *Group Fitness Instructor Manual*. Santiago, CA: American Council on Exercise, 2000.

Barlow, Wilfred. *The Alexander Principle*. London: Victor Gollancz Ltd., 1990.

Bean, Anita. "Protein the Powerhouse." *Fitpro*, Feb./March 2001.

Berk, Lotte, and Prince, Jean. *The Lotte Berk Method of Exercise*. London: Quartet Books, 1978.

Bingham, Sheila. *Dictionary of Nutrition: A Consumer's Guide to the Facts of Food*. London: Barrie and Jenkins, 1977.

Bird, Steve. "Is Exercise Really Good for Us?" *Biologist*, vol. 44, no. 5, Nov. 1997.

Blakey, Paul. *The Muscle Book*. Starrord, UK: Bibliotek Books, 1992.

Brennan, Richard. *The Alexander Technique Workbook*. Shaftsbury, Dorset, UK: Element Books Ltd., 1998.

British Medical Association. *Complete Guide to Family Health Encyclopaedia*. London: Dorling Kindersley, 1995.

Cook, Simon, and Toms, Tony. *Royal Marine Commando Exercises*. London: Sphere Books Ltd., 1990.

Cullum, Rodney, and Mowbray, Lesley. *The English YMCA Guide to Exercise to Music*. London: Pelham Books, 1992.

Donovan, Grant; McNamara, Jane; and Gianoli, Peter. *Exercise Danger*. Floreat Park, Western Australia: Wellness Australia Pty. Ltd., 1988.

Egger, Gary, and Champion, Nigel, eds. *The Fitness Leader's Handbook*, 3rd ed. Kenthurst, Australia: Kangaroo Press, 1997.

Fair, John D. "Isometrics or Steroids? Exploring New Frontiers of Strength in the Early 1960s." *Journal of Sports History*, Spring 1993, 20(1): 1–24.

Food and Agriculture Organization of the UN. *Joint FAO/WHO Expert Consultation on Human Vitamin and Mineral Requirements*. 21–30 September 1998 (revised July 2000), Rome: Food and Agriculture Organization of the UN.

Fox, Stuart Ira. *Human Physiology*, 5th ed. Dubuque, IA: Wm. C. Brown Publishers, 1996.

Gray, John. *Your Guide to the Alexander Technique*. New York: St. Martin's Press, 1991.

Hegarty, Vincent. *Nutrition, Food and the Environment*. St. Paul, MN: Eagan Press, 1995.

Hewett, James. *Yoga*. London: Hodder Headline, 1997.

Hicks, Andrew; McGill, Stuart; and Hughson, Richard. "Tissue Oxygenation by Near-Infrared Spectroscopy and Muscle Blood Flow During Isometric Contractions of the Forearm." *Canadian Journal of Applied Physiology*, 1999, 24(3).

Hughes, Joyce, ed. *Your Greatest Guide to Calories*. London: John Starr, 1980.

Kosich, Daniel. "Functional Kinesiology Movement Analysis." *Fitpro*, Oct./Nov. 2000.

Marchall, Janette, and Heughan, Anne. *Eat for Life Diet*. London: Vermillion, 1992.

McFarlane, Stewart. *The Complete Book of T'ai Chi*. London: Dorling Kindersley, 1997.

Mehta, Mira. *How to Use Yoga*. London: Lorenz Books, 1994.

Menezes, Allan. *Complete Guide to Joseph H. Pilates' Techniques of Physical Conditioning*. Alameda, CA: Hunter House, 2000.

Ministry of Agriculture, Fisheries and Food. *Manual of Nutrition*, 10th ed., London: The Stationary Office Books, 1995.

New Encyclopedia Brittanica, Macropaedia, 15th ed., s.v. "Human Evolution."

Newsholme, Eric; Leech, Tony; and Duester, Glenda. *Keep On Running: The Science of Training and Performance*. Chichester, UK: John Wiley and Sons, 1994.

Pawlett, Raymond. *T'ai Chi: A Practical Introduction*. San Diego, CA: Thunder Bay Press, 1999.

Peeke, Pamela. "When Stress Makes You Fat." *Fitpro*. Aug./Sept. 2000.

Pinckney, Callan. *Callanetics Countdown*. London: Ebury Press, 1990.

Reader's Digest. *Good Health Fact Book*. London: Reader's Digest Association, 1999.

————. *Foods That Harm, Foods That Heal: An A–Z Guide to Safe and Healthy Eating*. London: Reader's Digest Association, 1997.

Robinson, Lynne, and Thomson, Gordon. *Pilates*. London: Pan Books, 1999.

Robinson, Lynne; Fisher, Helge; Knox, Jacqueline; and Thomson, Gordon. *The Official Body Control Pilates Manual*. London: Macmillan Publishers Ltd., 2000.

Rosser, Mo. *Body Fitness and Exercise: Basic Theory and Practice for Therapists*. London: Hodder and Stoughton, 1999.

Schulze, Sonja. "Managing Patello-Femoral Pain." *Fitness Network*, June/July 2000.

Shave, Robert, and Whyte, Greg. "Can the Heart Fatigue?" *Fitpro*, Aug./Sept. 2000.

Smith, Tony, ed. *The Human Body*. London: Dorling Kindersley, 1995.

Stewart, Mary. *Yoga*. New York: McGraw-Hill, 1998.

————. *Yoga Over 50*. New York: Fireside, 1994.

Stroud, Mike. *Survival of the Fittest: Understanding Health and Peak Physical Performance*. London: Random House, 1998.

Troop, Nick, and Seato, Steven. *The Handbook of Running*. London: Pelham Books, 1997.

Williams, Peter L., et al., eds. *Gray's Anatomy*, 37th ed. London: Churchill Livingston, 1989.

Additional Resources: Selected Useful Websites

www.bmb.leeds.ac.uk/illingworth/muscle
The website of the School of Biochemistry and Molecular Biology, University of Leeds, contains detailed and well-illustrated explanations of the structure of muscles and their function.

www.eatright.org
The American Dietetic Association website provides good and extensive coverage of the nutritional contents of different foods and includes information on the special requirements for the elderly.

www.mayoclinic.com
The Mayo Clinic website includes concise information on sports injuries and their causes and treatments.

www.meddean.luc.edu/lumen/MedEd/ GrossAnatomy/dissector/mml/ index.html
The website of the Loyola University Medical Education Network gives concise information on muscles, including their origin, insertion, nerve supply, and action.

www.nismat.org/index.html
Created by the Nicholas Institute of Sports Medicine and Athletic Trauma (NISMAT) at Lenox Hill Hospital, New York, this website provides excellent coverage of exercise physiology, nutrition, and athletic training, as well as muscle contraction and energy supply.

www.nutrition.org.uk
The British Nutrition Foundation website provides useful data on nutrition in the United Kingdom.

www.pueblo.gsa.gov/press/nfcpubs/
The website of the Federal Communication Information Center offers a wide range of articles, including several on health, nutrition, and related topics.

www.runnersworld.co.uk/injury/ injury2.html
This website is a good information source for sports injuries, especially those associated with running.

Index

A

abdominal exercises, Conventional Body Crunch, 103–104; Moon Walk, 109–110; Pelvic Floor Exercise, 110; Reverse Abdominal Squeeze, 107–108; Scaling the Wall, 211–212; for seniors, 210–213; Shoulder to Knee, 111–112; Side Reaches, 110–111; Transverse Abdominal Squeeze, 105–106; Wall Walk, 212–213; "Z" Position, 112–113

abdominal muscles, 27–28; external obliques, 102, 103, 152; internal obliques, 102, 103, 152; rectus abdominus, 25–26, 86, 102, 103, 104, 151–152; structure of, 102; transverse abdominus, 102, 103, 105

abdominal stretches, Yawn, the, 151; "Z" Stretch, 152

abduction, 26

abductor muscles, 24, 29

Achilles tendon, 166, 167; injuries, 171

actin, 31, 32, 35

active stretching, 145–146

acupressure, 64

adduction, 26

adductor muscles, 24, 30; exercises for, 122–124; Groin Stretch, 156; injuries, 170;

stretching, 72, 156; Wide-Angle Stretch, 157

adenosine diphosphate (ADP), 41

adenosine triphosphate (ATP), 41, 43, 195

adipose (fat) tissue, 41, 51, 179

aerobic activity, 7, 69; advantages of, 75–76

aerobic energy system, 41–43

aerobic training, aerobic curve, 76–78, 80; benefits of, 75–76; circuits, 82–84; classes, 79–82; high-impact, 81–82; low-impact, 80–82; running, 78–79; for seniors, 208–209; target heart rate, 75

aging, 55–56, 207–226; and aerobics, 208–209; and arm muscles, 136–137; and back problems, 209–210; and benefits of exercise, 56, 207–209; and flexibility loss, 141–142; and muscle shortening, 9; and nutrition, 222–226; and osteoporosis, 20–21, 57; and strength training, 209–226

alcohol, 194, 205–206

Alexander, Frederick Matthias, 65, 66

Alexander Technique, 60, 65–67, 68, 91

alignment, body, 91–97

Allied Dunbar National Fitness Survey, 3

alpha-linolenic acid, 179

amenorrhea, 57

American Dietetic Association, 222

American Heart Association, 3–4, 182

amino acids, 184–186

anabolic process, 50

anaerobic energy system, 41, 43

anemia, megaloblastic, 203

anemia, pernicious, 203

aponeurosis, 103

appendicular skeleton, 17

arm exercises, Back Arm Lifts, 139; Scissoring the Arms, 139–140; Triceps Extension, 137–139

arm muscles, 136–140

arm stretches, 154

arthritis, 166, 169

atherosclerosis, 181, 201

axial skeleton, 17

B

back exercises; back extension, 114; latissimus dorsi, 135–136; for seniors, 213–214

back muscles, 113–114, 134–136

back pain, 170; in seniors, 209–210

back stretches, Feline Stretch, 148–149, 214; Forearm Twist, 154; Full Cobra, 151; Full Serpent, 150–151; Half Serpent, 149–150; Prayer Position, 149; Roll-Back, 153; Roll-Forward, 153–154; Standing Feline Stretch, 214–215

baker's cyst, 169

ballistic stretching, 144–145

basal metabolic rate (BMR), 41, 54; calculating, 49–50, 227–228

beauty, concept of, 2

beriberi, 199, 203

Berk, Lotte, 59, 91

beta-carotene, 199–200

biceps, 23–24, 26, 27; stretching, 154

blood clotting, 201

blood pressure, 14, 36, 38

blood sugar, 41. *See also* sugar

BMI. *See* body mass index (BMI)

BMR. *See* basal metabolic rate (BMR)

body fat, 13, 41; burning of, 43; spot reduction of, 54–55; storage, 51

body mass index (BMI), 11–13, 187; determining, 12

body shape, 47–49, 89; apple shape, 54–55; pear shape, 54–55

bone density, 20–21

bones, development of, 18–21; injuries, 166; types of, 18

Borg, Gunner, 8

breathing, 39–40; and *qi gong*, 163–164; techniques, 94–95, 100–101, 147–148. *See also* respiratory (pulmonary) system

bursitis, 166, 169

buttocks (gluteals) exercises, 114–124; Acute Angle Moving In, 120; Back Leg Lift, 115–117; Modified Buttock Lift, 120–122; Right-Angle Lift, 119; Sequential Contractions, 117–118; Side Leg Lift, 117; Straight Leg Extension, 118–119

buttocks (gluteals) stretches, Buttocks Stretch, 154–155; Hold the Horns, 155–156

C

calcium, 193–194, 200; requirements for seniors, 223

calf muscles, 131–132; stretching, 159–160

callanetics, 59, 91

calories, 40–41; daily intake, 52; defined, 229; requirements for athletes, 189

carbohydrate loading, 190–191

carbohydrates, 41, 178; food sources, 177; requirements for athletes, 189, 190

cardiac cycle, 38

cardiac muscle, 35–37

catabolic process, 50

chest exercises, Chest Press, 134; Push-Ups, 132–134

chi, 63–64

China, 63–65

chlorine, 194

cholesterol, 180, 181–183; recommended level, 182

chromium, 198

circuit training, 82–84

circulatory (cardiovascular) efficiency, 5, 7

circulatory system, 36

circumduction, 30

classes, fitness, 79–82

compartment syndrome, 90

conditioning, body, 85–98

constipation, 224–225

contraction, muscle, 86–90; static, 86–88; types of, 87

contusions, 166

copper, 196

core stability, 61, 92–97

cortisol, 41, 51, 54

creatine phosphate system, 44

cross-training, 173

D

deltoids, 24, 27, 136–137; stretching, 73, 154

diaphragm, 37, 39

diet, 51–54, 174–206; for athletes, 191; requirements for sports, 188–206; in U.S., 186–188

dietary patterns, 186–188

dieting, 53, 174–175

dorsi flexion, 30

Duester, Glenda, *xiv*

dynamic flexibility, 15

E

Eco-Challenge, 56

ectomorph, 48–49, 89

endomorph, 48–49, 89

endorphins, 54

endurance, 5, 6; assessment, 14–15; building, 101

energy, 40–41; expended in sports, 53

energy cycle, 42

energy systems, 40–45; aerobic, 41–43; anaerobic, 43; comparison of, 44; creatine phosphate, 44; and exercise, 45; lactate, 43–44

essential amino acids, 184

essential fatty acids (EFAs), 179

estimated average requirement (EAR), 52–53, 54

estrogen, 208

exercise, benefits of, *xiii*; FITTA (Frequency, Intensity, Time, Type, and Adherence) principle, 75; and seniors, 207–209; setting targets, 46–57; trends in, 58–60; weight-bearing, 21

extension, 26

extensor muscle, 23

F

facultative thermogenesis, 50

fartlek, 78

fat. *See* body fat

fats, dietary, 178–180, 187; recommended intake, 182–183

fatty acids, 41, 178–180

fiber, 178, 224

fitness assessment, 11–15; blood pressure, 14; body fat, 13; body mass index (BMI), 11–13; endurance, 14–15; flexibility, 15; height, 11–13; pulse rate, 13; stamina, 14–15; strength, 14; weight, 11–13

fitness, elements of, 5–7

fitness testing. *See* fitness assessment

FITTA (Frequency, Intensity, Time, Type, and Adherence) principle, 75, 90, 101

flexibility, 5, 6, 15

flexibility training, 141–164; exercises for the arms, 154; exercises for the buttocks, 154–157; exercises for the legs, 157–160; exercises for the torso, 148–154

flexion, 26; extreme, 147, 172

flexor muscle, 23–24

Food and Agriculture Organization (FAO), 53

Food Guide Pyramid, 175, 176, 183, 187, 188

foods, caloric content, 52; cholesterol content, 180; for seniors, 225. *See also* Food Guide Pyramid; nutrition

fractures, 166, 170

free radicals, 197

Funk, Casimir, 199

fusion fitness, and breathing technique, 100–101; compared with Pilates, 97; evolution of, 98

and importance of posture, 91–97; principles of, 68–69, 90–97

G

gender differences and exercise, 56–57

genetics and body type, 47

glucose, 41

gluteus maximus, 29, 31, 114–124

glycemic index, 189–190

glycogen, 41, 178

glycogen loading, 190

glycolysis, 41, 43

goals, exercise, 46–57

Golgi tendon organs, 33

H

hamstring test, 15–16

hamstrings, 30, 161–163; exercise, 129–131; injuries, 170; stretching, 72

hatha yoga, 60, 61

HDL cholesterol, 181–182

heart rate, 7, 36; raising, 72

high-impact aerobics, 81–82

holistic exercise, 60–68, 90–91; advantages of, 91; and aerobics, 67–68; Alexander Technique, 65–67, 68; disadvantages of, 90–91; Pilates, 67, 68; *t'ai chi chuan*, 63–65; yoga, 60–63, 68

hormones, and bone development, 20; cortisol, 41, 51, 54; estrogen, 208; noradrenaline, 204; production of, 198; thyroid, 196

hypercalcemia, 200
hyperplasia, 51
hypertension, 36, 38
hypertrophy, 51

I

iliopsoas, 93
injuries, 165–173; bones, 166; joints, 166; ligaments, 168; muscles, 166–167; tendons, 167; treatment of, 173
International Olympic Committee, 191
inverted poses (yoga), 61–63
iodine, 196
isometric training, 59–60, 86–88
isotonic training, 86

J

jazzercise, 79–82
joint capsule, 22
joint receptors, 33
joints, ball-and-socket, 21–22; ellipsoidal, 21; hinge, 21; injuries to, 166; mobile (movable), 21; mobilizing (warm-up), 71–72; partially movable, 21; pivot, 21; types of, 22
Joule, J. P., 40
joules, 40, 229

K

Karvonen formula, 7
Keep on Running (Newsholme, Leech, and Duester), xiv
kickboxing, 79–82

Klein, Helen, 56, 216
Krebs cycle, 42
Krebs, Hans, 42
kwashiorkor, 184
kyphosis, 19

L

lactate system, 43–44
lactic acid, 43
lactose intolerance, 223–224
latissimus dorsi, 25, 29, 135–136, 153–154; stretching, 148–151
LDL cholesterol, 181–182
Leech, Tony, xiv
leg exercises, Back Leg Lift, 217–218; Barre, the, 128–129; Conventional Squats, 124–125; Full Flight, 161–162; Heel Raises, 131–132; Inner Thigh Seesaw, 122–124; Leg Curl, 130–131, 218–219; Pedal and Stride, 126–128; Side Leg Lift, 219–220; Squats with Support, 215–216
leg stretches, 154–161; Calf Muscle, 159–160; Calf Stretch Using Wall, 220–221; Forward-Bend Stretch, 158–159; Hamstring Stretch Using Wall, 221–222; Stretching in Flight, 161; Thigh and Shin-Muscle Stretch, 157–158; Thigh Stretch with Support, 216
ligaments, 21; injuries, 168
linoleic acid, 179
lipoproteins, 181
lordosis, 19

low-impact aerobics, 80–82
lung capacity, 40

M

macrominerals, calcium, 193–194; chlorine, 194; magnesium, 194; phosphorus, 194–195; potassium, 195; sodium, 195–196
magnesium, 194
manganese, 198
marathons, 79
medical check-up, importance of, 9, 15
menopause, 208
mesomorph, 48–49, 89
metabolic rate, 50
metabolism, 50
microminerals, chromium, 198; copper, 196; iodine, 196; iron, 196–197; manganese, 198; molybdenum, 198; selenium, 197; sulfur, 198; zinc, 197–198
minerals, 192–198; macrominerals, 193–196; microminerals, 196–198; recommended daily intake, 192
mitochondria, 42
molybdenum, 198
monounsaturated fatty acids, 179
motor skills, 5, 6–7
muscle, 23–37, 86–90; abductors, 24; actions of, 26, 30; adductors, 24; cardiac, 23, 35–37; contraction of, 31; depressors, 25; extensor, 23; flexor, 23–24;

involuntary, 23; levators, 25; opposing-muscle groups, 89; principles of contraction, 86–90; skeletal, 23–35; smooth, 23, 35; sphincter, 25; striated, 23, 31; structure of, 35; synergist, 25; voluntary, 23. *See also specific muscles*

muscle fibers, 30–35; fast-twitch, 34–35; slow-twitch, 34–35

muscle injuries, 166–167

muscle spindles, 33

music and exercise, 101, 102, 163, 210

myocardial contractions, 36

myocardium, 35–37

myofibrils, 31, 32

myosin, 31, 32, 35

N

National Institutes of Health, 51

neuromuscular (muscle) spindles, 33

Newsholme, Eric, *xiv*

noradrenaline, 204

nutrition, 51–54, 174–206; carbohydrates, 177, 178; and cholesterol, 180, 181–183, 182; effects on body shape, 47; fats, 178–180; fatty acids, 178–180; fiber, 178; Food Guide Pyramid, 175, 176; and minerals, 192–198; and proteins, 183–186; salt intake, 194, 195–196; for seniors, 222–226; and sports, 188–206; sugar,

178; in the U.S., 186–188; and vitamins, 198–204; water requirements, 204–205

O

obesity, 3

Olympic Games, *xii*, 2–3

osteoblasts, 20

osteoclasts, 20

osteomalacia, 200

osteoporosis, 20–21, 57, 210

overload, 8, 84, 171

overtraining, 84

P

Patanjali, 60

pectorals, 24, 27; exercises for, 132–134, 153–154

Peeke, Pamela, 51

pellagra, 203

pelvic floor exercise, 110, 213

pelvic tilt, 96

pentathlon, *xii*

perceived exertion rate, 8, 9

periosteum, 21

personal maximum heart rate, 7, 77

phosphate, 41

phosphorus, 194–195

Pilates, 60, 61, 67, 68, 96

Pilates, Joseph H., 67

Pinckney, Callan, 59

plantar flexion, 30

point of insertion (muscle), 23, 25

point of origin (muscle), 23, 25

polyunsaturated fatty acids, 179

position, exercise, 99–100

posture, 91–97, 142

potassium, 195

pregnancy, 105

pronation, 30, 172

proprioceptive neuromuscular facilitation (PNF), 146

proprioceptors, 33, 34

proteins, 183–186; intake of, 185; requirements for athletes, 191; requirements for seniors, 222

pulse, 7, 13, 36; raising, 72

push-ups, 86, 172

Q

qi gong, 64, 95; breathing techniques, 163–164

quadriceps, 29, 124–129; injuries, 170; in seniors, 215–216; stretching, 73, 157–158. *See also* thigh exercises

quadriceps test, 15–16

R

race, and body type, 47–48

raja yoga, 60–61

recommended daily allowance (RDA), 52–53, 54

recti breathing, 61

relaxation, 163

repetition of exercise (reps), 101–102

resistance, body, 90–97

respiratory efficiency, 5

respiratory (pulmonary) system, 37–40

rest, importance of, 84, 171

rhomboids, 28, 134–135

RICE (rest, ice, compression, and elevation), 173

rickets, 200

runner's knee, 166, 169

running, 78–79

S

safety, 168, 171–173

salt, 187, 194, 195–196, 224

sarcomere, 31, 32

saturated fatty acids, 179, 182, 224

screening questionnaire, 9–10

scurvy, 199

selenium, 197

seniors, and aerobics, 208–209; exercises for, 209–222; and nutrition, 222–226; and strength training, 209

serotonin, 204

serving size, 176

shin muscles, 131–132

shin splints, 90, 166, 173

shoulder test, 15–16

sit-and-reach test, 15–16

sit-ups, 25–26, 86, 88

skeletal muscle, 23–35; abductors, 24; adductors, 24; depressors, 25; extensor, 23; flexor, 23–24; latissimus dorsi, 25; levators, 25; sphincter, 25; synergist, 25

skeleton, 17–22; bones, development of, 18–21; bones,

types of, 18; joints, 21–22; spinal column, 19

smooth muscle, 35

sodium, 195

somatotype, 47–49

sphincter muscles, 25

spinal column, 19; stabilizing, 92–97

sprains, 165, 169

spurs, 166, 170

stamina, 14–15

starch, 178

static flexibility, 15

static stretching, 145

step aerobics, 79–82

step test, 14–15

stomach crunches, 25–26, 86

strains, 165

strength, 5, 6, 14; building, 101

strength training, 55; for seniors, 209–226

stress, and appetite, 51

stretch reflex, 144

stretches, for the arms, 154; for the buttocks, 154–157; for the legs, 157–160; for the torso, 148–154

stretching, active, 145–146; after exercise, 34, 220; ballistic, 144–145; benefits of, 142–143; developmental, 144; preparatory, 9, 70–74, 144, 147, 173; progression in training, 160–163; proprioceptive neuromuscular facilitation (PNF), 146; static, 145; types of, 143–146

striated muscle. *See* skeletal muscle

Stroud, Mike, 56

sugar, 178, 187; and seniors, 224

sulfur, 198

supination, 30

Survival of the Fittest (Stroud), 56

synergist muscles, 25

synovial membrane, 22

synovitis, 169

T

t'ai chi chuan, 60, 63–65, 94

tan tien, 64, 94

target heart rate, 7

tendonitis, 167, 171

tendons, 21

thigh exercises, Barre, the, 128–129; Conventional Squats, 124–125; Inner Thigh Seesaw, 122–124; Pedal and Stride, 126–128

thyroid gland, 196

trace elements. *See* microminerals

training programs, sample, 230–241

trapezius, 28, 134–135, 153–154

treadmills, 79

triceps, 23, 26, 27, 31, 137–140; stretching, 73, 154

triglycerides, 179

U

unsaturated fatty acids, 179

U.S. Food and Nutrition Board, 194, 195

V

vertebrae, 19

vitamins, 198–204; fat-soluble, 199–201; recommended daily intake, 202; requirements for seniors, 224; vitamin A (retinol), 199–200; vitamin B complex, 201, 203–204; vitamin C, 204; vitamin D, 200; vitamin E, 201; vitamin K, 201; water-soluble, 201–204

W

waist, exercises for, 110–113

warm-up, 9, 22–23, 70–74; benefits of, 74

water, required intake, 204–205; for seniors, 224

weights, 89

women and exercise, 1–3, 56–57

World Health Organization (WHO), on alcohol consumption, 205; and body mass index, 13; classification of blood pressure, 14; and nutrition, 53, 175, 176, 187

Y

yoga, 1, 60–63, 68; dog pose, 63; and inverted postures, 62; peacock pose, 62–63

Z

Z-band, 32

zinc, 197–198

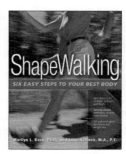
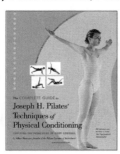
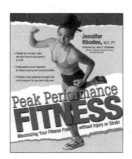

ORDER FORM

NAME

ADDRESS

CITY/STATE   ZIP/POSTCODE

PHONE   COUNTRY (outside of U.S.)

TITLE	QTY	PRICE	TOTAL
Fusion Fitness (paperback)		@ $17.95	
Fusion Fitness (hardcover)		@ $29.95	
Prices subject to change without notice			

Please list other titles below:

		@ $	
		@ $	
		@ $	
		@ $	
		@ $	

Check here to receive our book catalog ❑   *FREE*

Shipping Costs:
By Priority Mail, first book $4.50, each additional book $1.00
By UPS and to Canada, first book $5.50, each additional book $1.50
For rush orders and other countries call us at (510) 865-5282

TOTAL
Less discount @ _____ %
TOTAL COST OF BOOKS
Calif. residents add 7½ sales tax
add Shipping & handling
TOTAL ENCLOSED
Please pay in U.S. funds only

(_____)

❑ Check ❑ Money Order ❑ Visa ❑ MasterCard ❑ Discover

Card # _____ Exp. date _____

Signature _____

Complete and mail to:

Hunter House Inc., Publishers
PO Box 2914, Alameda CA 94501-0914
Phone (510) 865-5282 Fax (510) 865-4295
You can also order by calling **(800) 266-5592**
of from **www.hunterhouse.com**

FUF 3/2003